Qualit

Nurs

C000195486

Quality Assurance
in
Nursing Practice

Nan Kemp
RGN, RCNT, Dip N (Lond)
*Freelance Nurse Consultant for Quality
Assurance and the Nursing Process*

Eileen W. Richardson
RGN, SCM, RNT, BA, MA
*Divisional Head (Adult Branch) Dorset and Salisbury
College of Midwifery and Nursing*

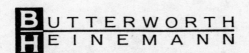

Heinemann Medical
An imprint of Butterworth–Heinemann Ltd
Halley Court, Jordan Hill, Oxford OX2 8EJ

PART OF REED INTERNATIONAL BOOKS

LONDON GUILDFORD OXFORD BOSTON SINGAPORE
SYDNEY TOKYO TORONTO WELLINGTON

First published 1990

British Library Cataloguing in Publication Data
Kemp, Nan
    Quality assurance in nursing practice.
    1. Medicine. Nursing. Quality assurance
    I. Title.   II. Richardson, Eileen W.
    610.730685

ISBN 0 7506 0019 5

Printed and bound in Great Britain by
Biddles Ltd, Guildford and Kings Lynn

Contents

Acknowledgements

To Dr Derek Browne, of Brockenhurst, who believes in holistic medicine, gives quality care, and without whose support and encouragement this book would never have been written.

To three nurses who took time and trouble to read and critique the manuscript, we are deeply grateful to: Pam Grosvenor, Portsmouth and South East Hampshire Health Authority. Caroline Waldman, The MacMillan Unit, Odstock Hospital, Salisbury and Denise Barnett, West Essex Health Authority.

To Nora Snowdon and Sarah Kemp for their patience and secretarial help. To the Butterworth–Heinemann staff; Susan Devlin and Helen Plows for their guidance and kindness. To the secretaries and telephonists for their courtesy.

We are grateful to the following people who courteously answered our questions and or provided information: Chris Naym, Bryan Wilson, Helen Kendall, Mary Pearce, Elizabeth Mason, Di Sale, Geraldine Padilla, Brenda Baxter, Nancy Cox, Jaqualine Flindall, Malcom McGreevy, Sue Nattress, Tony Pepper, Mary Angel, Alison Kitson and the staff of the Standards of Care project, Royal College of Nursing and the Institute of Nursing, Oxford.

The staff of the Quality Assurance Department – King's fund Centre. The staff of the Nursing Research Department, Department of Health. The staff of the Wessex Regional Health Authority Headquarters Library. Fiona Robson and staff of the Royal College of Nursing Library.

We are also grateful to all those people who gave us permission to use their work. Last but not least Bob and Sarah Kemp and Gillian and Nicholas Heslop for their encouragement and positive support.

Note to the reader

For the sake of clarity the pronoun 'she' refers to the nurse and on occasions 'he' refers to the patient. No bias is intended in the use of pronouns; we trust our readers will understand. Patient is used to refer to the client, resident or person receiving care.

Preface

Although there has always been a professional commitment to provide quality of nursing care, it is only recently that nurses have become interested in the construction of a system for the measurement of their practice. The National Health Service Management Inquiry report of 1983 found that, 'The NHS lacked any real continuous evaluation of performance against criteria.' The report brought change to the management hierarchy controlling health care. Nurses have become more vulnerable as a result; often now being asked to give account of their practice to non-nurse managers. There is more than ever a need for nurses to be able to work from a sound knowledge base if they are discussing nursing and other resource needs.

We felt that there was a need for a book that would be easily accessible to all those interested in quality for whatever reason. A book which would be easy for them to follow, but also one which collated information from a variety of sources.

In the book we start by giving background information about the development of quality assurance and put forward suggestions for the organization of a quality assurance programme for nursing. In Chapter 3 we focus on setting standards and criteria and the development of an instrument to measuring the quality of care. We highlight some of the difficulties this involves and offer suggestions to solve them. In Chapters 4, 5 and 6 we focus on measuring quality in the domain of structure, process and outcome respectively. We discuss quality monitoring methodologies and report on the debate about evaluating process versus outcome. We have included examples of standards which have been developed by nurses and others for clinical practice. In Chapter 7, the focus is on education and offers practical guidance to those involved in implementing quality assurance initiatives.

Often nurses are asked to introduce new systems without the educational support that would enable them to be more effective. We have used our backgrounds both in education and practice to address this problem. We have attempted to give information in a way which is easily understood and a range of knowledge which, although not exhaustive, brings together ideas from a number of people working in this field. We also hope we have gone some way to provide the skills needed to pass on this information to others.

Introduction

In all walks of professional life, nurses are being called to account for the standard of their practice. The United Kingdom Central Council for Nursing, Midwifery and Health Visiting (1989) state that 'the exercise of accountability requires the practitioner to seek to achieve and maintain high standards'. The purpose of this book is to try to help nurses to set standards of care and to do so in an organized and systematic way.

We are concerned that the care which nurses give can measure up to standards which have clearly been defined and agreed to. Caring must have 'quality' a concept that appears difficult to define. *Chambers Dictionary* (1980) states that 'quality is that which makes a thing what it is: nature, character, attitude: grade of goodness: excellence'. How can we conceptualize such a definition? Many thinkers have found difficulty in isolating quality sufficiently to describe it. In the book *Zen and the Art of Motorcycle Maintenance* we find Pirsig, (1987) spending many chapters wrestling with the idea. In the end he claims it was incapable of definition. He understands it as a driving force within us which impels us to seek improvement; a special kind of growing level of awareness that differs between individuals. And without which 'life would just be living without any value or purpose at all'.

In his autobiography, Marcus Sieff (1988), the President of Marks and Spencer described his first encounter with quality in a much more practical way. He was staying in a Manchester hotel with his Uncle Simon who ordered a kipper for his breakfast. It duly arrived beautifully presented on a silver salver. His uncle tasted it and sent it back. It was only on receipt of the third kipper that he said 'That tastes good. That is quality.'

At a conference in 1986 Penny Prophit spoke about 'the pur-.

suit of excellence involving the recognition that quality is a value and as a corporate vision requires the clarification of values through individual and personal journeys of discovery'.

Perhaps we can only conceive of quality in terms of the 'goodness' that is inherent in the object with which we are concerned. So that we need not struggle to conceive of quality in an abstract sense but learn to recognize it in our everyday experience.

Our everyday experiences as nurses demand we think of quality in terms of health care. There are those who have already attempted to do this, in defining quality one must define what the outcome of health should be. To quote the World Health Organization (WHO, 1986), 'Quality is . . . the comparison of how the level of care actually provided compares with that which is defined as the wanted level of care.' They suggest that 'the wanted level of care' is often a political decision and is calculated at the level above which care would be costly and below which it would be dangerous. It is to be hoped that such political decisions take into account the wishes and advice of health care providers and consumers.

Wilson Barnett (1981) described quality as 'referring to the value or benefit derived from care' and defines it as 'the degree of success achieved in reaching these goals' and therefore assumes 'an evaluation of care'. What do we mean when we say we are evaluating care? In simple language it usually means measuring how far the actual outcome of care prescribed has met the 'expected' outcomes for the client.

Quality Assurance in Nursing is about assuring the clients of the quality of the nursing care they are given. When we evaluate care we want to be able to measure how the care we have given compares with the standards we have set. Then we will have some recognizable yardstick with which to measure the quality of what we do.

References

MacDonald A. M. ed. (1980). *Chambers Dictionary* Edinburgh: Chambers.

Pirsig R. M. (1987) *Zen and the Art of Motorcycle Maintenance*. London: Corgi books.

Prophit P. (1986) Foreword to Quest for Quality; Proceedings of the 20th Annual Study Day of the Nursing Studies Association, University of Edinburgh.

Sieff M. (1988) *Don't Ask the Price*, London: Fontana, William Collins.

United Kingdom Central Council (1989) *Exercising Accountability*. London: U.K.C.C.

Wilson Barnett J. (1981) Janforum, *Journal of Advanced Nursing*. **6**, 503–14

World Health Organisation (March, 1986) *Nursing/Midwifery in Europe*, WHO Regional Unit for Europe.

Yura H., Walsh M. B. (1978) *The Nursing Process* 3rd edn. Norwalk: Appleton-Century-Crofts

1
The development of quality assurance

It is generally agreed that the first recorded account of any systematic study of nursing and health care was done by Florence Nightingale during her time in the Crimea. When she returned to this country she became more involved in nursing and in nurse training. In her *Notes on Nursing* (1858), we find quoted innumerable statements which relate to quality of care, one such example is 'unnecessary noise is the most cruel absence of care which can be inflicted, on sick or well'.

In North America the setting up of the Joint Commission on Accreditation of Hospitals (JCAH), was a landmark in the work towards the setting of acceptable standards of health care. Accreditation is a recognition of a hospital's compliance with established standards. JCAH developed from the Hospital Standardization Programme established in 1918 by the American College of Surgeons whose aim at that time was to develop a uniform medical record to ensure accuracy of clinical recording. One of the JCAH tasks is to survey hospitals, measuring performance against standards at the request of hospitals wishing accreditation. Subsequently this body has been a major influence in the development of quality assurance programmes in America. Its main purpose being to work towards the attainment of uniformly high standards within health care institutions.

Although this initiative in standard setting seems to have been taken by health care personnel in North America, British nurses too have continued to be concerned about the quality of the care they are giving. Caring is, after all, central to the practice of nursing.

During the 1960s in the United Kingdom there was concern about the quality of care as a result of adverse publicity generated by the publication of books such as *What's Wrong with Hospitals?* (Cohens, 1964) and *Sans Everything* (Robb, 1967). Professor Revans (1964), in his book *Standards for Morale* indicated that some inherent quality might determine both the patients recovery time and turnover of staff. Until this time no studies had been done which recommended the development of objective standards or criteria of quality (Baly, 1974). The Department of Health and Social Security (DHSS) expressed its concern by sponsoring a research project in the Education Department of the Royal College of Nursing (RCN) whose specific remit included: 'to develop techniques for measuring the quality of nursing care'. An account of the setting up of this project and the theoretical problems surrounding the establishment of criteria of quality of nursing care was published by the RCN in 1970 in the book entitled *The Proper Study Of The Nurse* by Professor McFarlane. This was subsequently followed by the selection of a wide range of topics for research. However McFarlane (1979) referring to the summary by Inmans points out that 'because the studies were so widely dispersed it is not possible to build the criteria measures into a scale, but the publication of the reports has made a major contribution to the quality of nursing care in that nurses are alerted to practices which result in poor quality nursing care and some potential criteria for quality are now available.'

Later in the 1970s underlying the need to encourage nurses to consider their professional standards, a series of letters were sent by the Chief Nursing Officer at the DHSS to all regional, area and district chief nurses. The purpose being to focus professional attention and promote discussion on one particular aspect of nursing at a time.

In 1978, the RCN set up a working committee on standards of nursing care which brought out its first report in 1979. This was followed in 1981 by the committee's second report entitled *Towards Standards*. One of the points the committee made at this stage was that the nurse should take it upon herself to use the framework of the nursing process to set the standards for her own patients in the light of their needs and her situation. In doing so she as an individual 'should accept accountability for her individual nursing action'.

At the same time WHO was working to similar ends. In 1984 the European region of the WHO published *Targets for Health for All*. This setting of targets provides a challenge and commitment to all member states to reduce inequalities in health. In so doing, it gives fuel to the debate on national health policies. Of particular pertinence is target 31 which states 'By 1990 all member states should have built effective mechanisms for ensuring quality of patient care within their health care systems'. In elaborating on this statement they stress the need to move beyond the measuring of the level of technical developments to ensuring that the health services of a country 'meet a variety of needs in an integrated way'. They stress the need for services to be both appropriate and acceptable to the consumer – a point worth underlining when considering the increased awareness of the consumer in this country.

It is also important to note their reference to the health care provided and the way in which a quality assurance programme should enable the individual to achieve constant self-improvement by the feedback he receives. It is also necessary to include an educational component into the health care worker's programme which specifically relates to 'the question of the quality of the service being provided and its acceptability to patients and their relatives'.

The implications for nursing/midwifery of the *Targets for Health for All* paper is discussed in a further WHO publication brought out in 1986. In relation to quality it states that 'Nurses and midwives should participate in the evaluation of care ... need to involve patients in decisions about their care and help them make informed choices by supplying them with the necessary information.'

They also add the important reminder to nurses that if they do not develop and apply their own standards they will be handed standards of practice from another discipline.

In February 1983, Norman Fowler who was then the Secretary of State at the DHSS set up the National Health Service (NHS) Management inquiry. The Chairman of the inquiry team Roy Griffiths, reported to the Secretary in October of the same year. This report subsequently known as 'the Griffiths Report', has had considerable impact on the NHS management and its philosophy and, as a result, on nursing. In an examination of the NHS at the time, the report states that 'it still lacks any real continuous evaluation of its performance against criteria'. There is a real need to evaluate performance because as we stated earlier we owe our clients value in the service we provide. In giving advice to the secretary the Griffiths team describes the NHS as 'a caring quality service, which has to balance the interests of the patient, the community, the taxpayer and the employees'. Its most important recommendation was that of introducing the general management process into the service – this meant the drawing together in one person responsibility for planning, implementation and control of performance.

The impact of general management on nursing has been quite considerable, not least in the resulting loss of a guaranteed nursing place in the management team and with it nursing's power to influence change. Management has a responsibility for ensuring quality of health care across the health district, but each professional group has a role and responsibility for setting its own standards within the district framework. In some districts the quality assurance management role has been taken across the board and in this way has deflected nursing from its original concern to evaluate its own service to patients. We pose the question is this a bad thing?

The changing role of nurses in management is a theme taken up by the seminar set up by the nursing division of the DHSS in April 1986. This seminar also identified as a major issue 'the nature of evaluation, autonomy and accountability in nursing as patterns of treatment change and nursing care of patients becomes more individualized'. Anne Poole, the Chief Nurse underlines the need for quality control when she says that nursing can no longer rely on intuition to determine whether its practice is effective. The time has come when we have to develop methods of measuring quality and effectiveness. Throughout the seminar, speakers emphasized the need to determine effectiveness of care and quality in practice. As a result of the seminar 'A strategy for action' was drawn up. This included as one of the identified issues, 'The management of nursing practice in relation to the determination of standards and the assessment of quality assurance.'

In 1979 the Nurses, Midwives and Health Visitors Act provided the profession with the opportunity through the United Kingdom Central Council for Nursing, Midwifery and Health Visiting, (UKCC) to lay down a code of conduct for the professional. In its revised version published in 1984 emphasis is placed on the individual's accountability for her own decisions and actions. There is a recognized relationship between accountability and standards of practice. We will indicate in Chapter 2 how before setting standards the philosophy of nursing must be identified. Once this is done the standards will be seen to hold the values inherent in the philosophy. Nurses must be given the necessary education to develop the competence to practise to the accepted standard. It is this level of competence for which the practitioner is responsible.

The 1979 Act also determined the need to change the 'Nurses Rules' and in 1983 a new 'Nurses, Midwives and Health Visitors Approval Order' was published. In Rule 18, the competencies required of someone who is eligible to be admitted to Parts 1, 3, 5 and 8 of the Register are given. These competencies include at (g) 'to review the effectiveness of the nursing care provided and where appropriate, initiate action which may be required'. We have previously said that the time has indeed come when nurses must be able to measure the effectiveness of their care.

The professional bodies have not been slow to add their weight to the question of quality. In 1985 the Royal College of Nursing Standards of Care project was set up and Dr Alison Kitson appointed as its leader. This followed on from the earlier work of their working committee on standards. The project will carry out research to establish the academic background to quality of care but will also 'spread the word with practical help and guidelines to grip the hearts and minds of every nurse in the country', (Kitson, 1985).

In the Autumn of 1987 the RCN produced a position statement on nursing entitled *In Pursuit of Excellence*. The steering group which devised this statement set themselves the task of defining 'a clear precise declaration of the values to which the profession sets itself'. The three main principles for nursing which the group identified were: equity, respect for persons and caring. Having identified the central beliefs about nursing in society they go on to provide nine statements as 'pointers to help nurses move towards providing a quality service' based on core concepts. Statement 4 is particularly relevant. 'Society and the individual can hold the nursing profession accountable for the quality of the service it delivers. The nursing profession accepts the responsibility to be held accountable for the quality of its service.'

As nurses, not only are we influenced by the Department of Health, the world-wide organization of the WHO and our professional bodies but also by the voice of the consumers. Surely their response to the service we are providing should be of paramount importance. We are more aware of them now both in the formal and informal organization and in their personal responses, but it was not always so!

In early discussions about NHS organizations in the 1960s there was no mention of the need for a consumer organization. We were used to laymen participating in management, committee and hospital boards but this was only by a selected few and no organization had been formed to take this on board. The consumers views were first specifically represented in the body referred to as 'the Community Health Council', but it was not until the passage of the 1973 NHS Reorganization Act that it officially came into being. These councils have played an important role in making the public's voice known to local health authorities. Most have been diligent in carrying out their function of 'reviewing the operation of the health service in its district and making recommendations for the improvement of such services'. The regulations also allow for such bodies to enter and inspect health authority premises and to make recommendations based on the findings of such visits. In later years the social acceptability of a health service to its clients has also been gauged by the useful surveys of patients and public satisfaction carried out by such bodies.

Many voluntary organizations are well established in the NHS and are often able to exert considerable pressure on the statutory bodies. Such organizations as Age Concern, MIND (National Association for Mental Health) and, NAWCH (National Association for the Welfare of Children in Hospital) are well known for the work that they have done in respect of those they represent. A good example of work such an organization has done is the NAWCH charter for Children in Hospital which was published in 1984 and sets standards for their care. This group has since gone on to produce a checklist for evaluating children's departments in hospitals.

Patients too have organized themselves into groups in order to have their voices heard. The Patients Association grew out of the indignation of one patient. An interesting comparison to this is the emergence in the community of 'patient participation groups' in general practice. These groups which are representative of those belonging to a practice meet regularly with the doctors and other practice staff in the interest of improving communication and the services. The Director of the recently established College of Health argues that the NHS can only make real progress when it finds out exactly what the consumer wants. She suggests that some of the things people do want are: not having to wait for a service they need, to be treated as a person, more information and help not to become patients (Rigg, 1985). These statements should not come as news to us, but it is worth reminding ourselves of their importance.

Information is more generally available to the public about individual health services. Women's magazines, daily newspapers or TV and radio have all from time to time given information and advice to the public. People's expectations of the services are now higher, they are more aware of their 'rights'. We must make sure that we listen to the voice of our consumers and take heed of what they are telling us. We have grown to expect praise and thanks from the grateful patient. How much do we know that their satisfaction is due to our care and how much to many other factors, including their own pleasure at leaving us to go home?

The Royal Commission on the Health Service which published its report *Patients' Attitudes to the Hospital Service* in 1978 found little dissatisfaction with the total services offered to people – 80% of inpatients thought the service was very good. Nevertheless when identifying some specific problem areas, two certainly gave cause for concern. Of adult patients, 43% felt they were woken too early, while 33% felt they were not given enough information about their progress. It is the latter area which is the most frequently quoted cause of patients' complaints both locally to health authorities and nationally to the Ombudsman.

Clearly there is room for improvement. The Griffiths report (1984) describes the consumer as 'a legitimate judge of quality' and suggests that market research techniques should be used 'to ascertain how well the service is being delivered to local level'. John Moore, then Secretary of State for Social Services, speaking in the Summer of 1988 reminds us that he believes 'that we must ensure that the customer is not only consulted but that his or her views are acted upon wherever possible'. We are part of those delivering service at local level. Let us be aware of the needs and wishes of our clientele and then make sure we are giving them the quality service they deserve. There are powerful forces telling us we should. We must listen not just to them but also to our own 'still small voice' of conscience.

As individuals we work within an organization. We must bring our individual expertise to share with our colleagues. In our next chapter we will be discussing the practical steps which are necessary to set up a quality assurance programme for nursing with the district.

References

Baly M. (1974) *Nursing and Social Change.* Oxford: Heinemann Medical Books.

Cohens G. (1964) *What's wrong with Hospitals?* Harmondsworth: Penguin.

Community Health Councils (1986) A Review of their Role and Structure. London: Community Health Council.

D.H.S.S. Strategy for Action (1986) Report of a Seminar held at DHSS. London: HMSO

Ham C. (1985) Consumerism in the N.H.S. – the State of the Art. *Health and Social Services Journal*, 30 May 1985.

Joint Commission on Accreditation of Hospitals (1982) Accreditation Manual for Hospitals. Chicago, USA: J.C.A.H.

Kitson A. (1985) *Standards of Care Project.* London: Royal College of Nursing.

McFarlane J. Prof. (1970) *The Proper Study of the Nurse.* London: Royal College of Nursing.

McFarlane J. Prof. (1980) Essays on Nursing. Working paper of the Royal commission on the N.H.S. No. RC2. London: King's Fund Centre

Moore J. (1988) Quality of Service – Patients as People, Speech to the Office of Health Economics, Seminar 5 July 1988.

NAWCH (1984) Charter for Children in Hospital. London: National Association for the Welfare of Children in Hospital.

National Health Service Management Inquiry Report (Griffiths, 1984) London: HMSO.

Nightingale F. (1858) *Notes on Nursing.* London: Harrison and Sons.

Revans R. W. (1964) *Standards for Morale: Cause and effect in hospitals.* Oxford: Nuffield Provincial Hospitals Trust.

Robb B. (1967) *Sans Everything: a case to answer.* London: Nelson.

Royal College of Nursing (1980) *Standards of Nursing Care.* London: Royal College of Nursing.

Royal College of Nursing (1981) *Towards Standards.* Report of a Working Party. London: Royal College of Nursing.

Royal College of Nursing (1987) *'In Pursuit of Excellence'.* Position Statement on Nursing. London: Royal College of Nursing.

Royal Commission on the National Health Service (1978) *Patients' Attitudes to the Hospital Service.* London: HMSO.

Rigg M. (1985) The customer's perspective. *Health and Social Services*

Journal. 30 May 1985

United Kingdom Central Council (1979) *Nurses, Midwives and Health Visitors Act.* London: HMSO.

United Kingdom Central Council (1983) *Nurses, Midwives and Health Visitors Approval Order.* London: HMSO.

World Health Organization (1984) *Targets for Health for All.* WHO, Regional Office for Europe.

World Health Organization (1986) *Targets for health for all: Implications for Nursing/Midwifery.* WHO, Regional Office for Europe.

2

Developing a quality assurance programme

In the previous chapter we discussed the reasons for evaluating the quality of care, we are now going on to discuss the setting up of a quality assurance programme. This can be defined as a 'planned and systematic approach to monitoring and evaluating the care provided (or service being delivered) that identifies opportunities for improvement and provides a mechanism through which action is taken to make and maintain these improvements'. *Australian Council on Hospital Standards – Educational Programme* (cited by Fitzgibbon, 1986).

In any health district there will be a committee with responsibility for coordinating and facilitating quality assurance activities at district level. Many health districts have in fact appointed a Director of Quality and in some instances this position has been taken by the most senior nurse in the organization, perhaps acknowledging the large and competent role nursing has in health care.

Below district level there is a very complex situation because individual groups at unit level and below may develop their own quality assurance programmes. These groups may belong to single disciplines or specialities such as medicine or surgery. We feel that in an ideal situation quality assurance groups should be multi-disciplinary.

Our focus is on a quality assurance programme for nursing although we feel that many of the principles we advocate can be applied to any quality assurance programme.

When the decision has been made to set up a quality assurance programme for nursing it is necessary that some form of steering group/working party is required.

Membership of the steering group

The group should include people with knowledge of the policies and resources of the district and of the District Quality Assurance Plan. It is essential that some members have experience and knowledge of the subject to be evaluated, there should also be a member from education for they have up-to-date knowledge about requirements of statutory bodies and can easily identify training needs and advise on how to meet these needs. It is also worth considering someone with counselling skills to help anticipate, prevent and work through any problems that may arise when such an innovation is introduced into work areas. The group should also have the facility to 'opt in' people with specialist knowledge; for example, a statistician to advise on measurement, and a nurse specialist when standards are being set in her particular area of expertise, for example, a stoma therapist.

It is interesting to note that a legal adviser is often a member of the steering group in some countries. One wonders when we will consider this necessary in the United Kingdom.

The chairperson of this group will probably be the person who reports to the District or Unit Quality Assurance Committee. It should be noted that to be effective the group should not be too large.

The role of the steering group

The major role of this group is the development of the Quality Assurance Programme together with the methodology to be used.

In order to do this an effective steering group consults and holds discussion with staff and others likely to be influenced by the undertaking. For nurses in the United Kingdom this may include the ethics committees, trade unions and professional organizations. It is often helpful to look at reports published by Community Health Councils and relevant patient organizations and voluntary bodies and consult them because they express the views of the community. If the patients are to be asked about their care in the course of monitoring quality, they should be informed and their permission should be sought before they are interviewed. Patient and visitor information sheets could aid this process, pointing out that the patient has a choice in whether or not to be interviewed and that anonymity is assured. Once this consultation process has taken place there are a series of steps which the group must undertake and will be discussed in the remainder of this chapter.

Before developing the programme and writing the plan this group must decide what are the purposes and objectives of the programme, examine the philosophy of its practice, and identify the resources available. Consideration must also be given to the intangible issues such as confidentiality (see Table 2.1).

Purpose

There will be a written statement of the purpose which is to enable an evaluation to take place of health care practices in a systematic manner. It should reinforce good practice, and identify problems leading to the implementation of a plan of action that will bring about a correction of these deficiencies, whilst at the same time giving support to all those involved.

Philosophy

In developing a quality assurance programme for nursing it is essential that the members of the group look at what nursing means to them as individuals and also as members of a group, in particular the approach to standards of care and the evaluation of nursing.

But what is the meaning of philosophy? *Chambers Dictionary* defines philosophy as 'pursuit of wisdom and knowledge'. Griffin (1980) sees philosophy 'as a thinking activity to increase knowledge and understanding about the world and about ourselves'.

To define and write a philosophy will call for much heart searching and debate: it is necessary but it may be uncomfortable. Chapman (1978) says 'the mental effort required to determine one's philosophy regarding any topic is time well spent'. Before clarifying and writing down our beliefs the questions should be asked 'What does nursing mean to us? Why are we doing what we are doing? Why should we spend so much effort in developing a quality assurance programme?' Some obvious answers that may be facetiously given are 'we have no choice', 'we've been sent' and 'it's policy'. These must also be explored.

Table 2.1 FLOW CHART TO DEMONSTRATE THE DEVELOPMENT OF A QUALITY ASSURANCE PROGRAMME FOR NURSING.

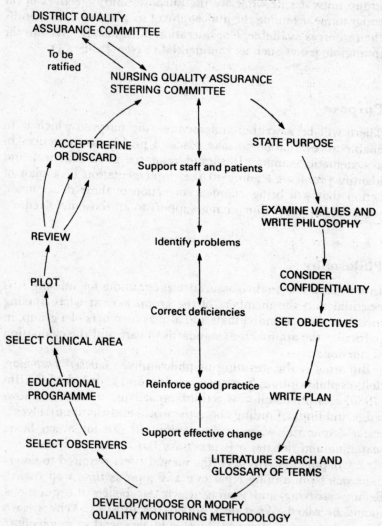

It may be that a particular department has relevant procedures and policies well thought out – nonetheless a philosophical statement is still required. Our procedures and policies should of course reflect our philosophy. This has to be the essential starting point because one needs to acknowledge different cultural and social norms, the requirements for education and the rights of the individual to choice, privacy and independence, self-esteem, identity, and worth.

If all this seems too daunting a task, it should be remembered that a philosophical statement well thought out will demonstrate a commitment to nursing and indicate our values to staff, patients and the society in which we live. MacFarlane (1982) says 'There is I believe a great need to preserve and use human values in health care, to reduce de-personalization, isolation and neglect of individuals, but also to develop and use scientific values and competence especially in nursing.' This would seem to epitomize what a quality assurance programme is all about.

Confidentiality

Increasingly these days information is being collected in the Health Service both about patients and about the service with which they are being provided. What is done with this information and who has access to it is a sensitive issue and one which must be discussed by the group at an early stage in their deliberations.

In the *Journal of Medical Ethics*, Phelby (1982) has spoken of the great anxiety which has resulted from the growth of the collection of data relating to individual patients for statistical purposes. There is a risk here to the health professional/client relationship if confidentiality seems to be imperilled.

The findings of quality assurance programmes do not name the patient or individual staff member whose care and work is being evaluated. However there has to be a means of identifying the ward or department from which the data came. This is necessary in order for the ward or department to retrieve findings of monitoring procedures. On the face of it, it would seem that information should either be disclosed publicly or not, but there are also degrees to which this can be done. Too many restrictions can serve as a barrier to evaluation and research and this may present difficulties when summarizing findings, writing reports and where there is a need for decisions to be made which will improve clinical practice. All these aspects must be borne in mind when those controlling quality assurance programmes are deciding a strategy.

Objectives

Setting the objectives for the programme is essential for these will act as a guide to progress. Those setting the objectives must be cognisant of the philosophy and resources of the district and its units.

The objectives must be realistic with regard to time and resources available and most important they should be appropriate for the people they are going to affect. It may be planned to ask a range and type of questions which patients have neither the physical or emotional strength to deal with. Demands may be made on staff for which they do not have the necessary skills.

Once these issues have been dealt with by the group it is necessary that they should devise the Quality Assurance Plan.

The plan

Any written plan that aims to bring about change should be concise, clearly understood, not too long and very importantly available to all those involved in an effort to aid communications, reduce stress and aid the successful implementation of the programme.

The quality assurance plan defines in writing the nursing strategy for implementing the quality assurance programme to cover all appropriate areas. It should contain the purpose of the programme which reinforces the Health Authority's commitment to a quality assurance programme and the group's philosophy as previously described. It is also wise to write the definition of a quality assurance programme into the plan for, as when looking at the purpose, it makes the people writing the plan and reading it think about what they are doing, why they are doing it, and whether indeed it is actually feasible. It identifies the role of the Quality Assurance Group and the objectives set by its members. The methodology to be used in assessing quality will be included if a decision has been made about this when the plan is written.

The plan must also identify those who are accountable and responsible for quality assurance initiatives. The plan should contain a description of the communication channels and the accountability pathways.

If a quality assurance coordinator is employed his or her job description may be attached to the quality assurance plan. Within the plan must also be the method to be used to evaluate the programme, and when this will be done. In North America this is usually done annually. Mention may also be made of how the findings will be processed and how frequently reports will be sent to the District Quality Assurance Committee and the appropriate managers.

The plan must have a timetable for the implementation of the programme; it is not sufficient that this be written within the objectives for there is a danger that it may get lost. A statement should be made as to the resources available, including costing and some reference to education should also be made.

There are certain elements of this plan which need further elaboration.

Cost

Setting up a quality assurance programme will inevitably incur costs. At this time of financial stringency in the NHS there is inevitably competition for scarce resources but it is essential that there is budgeting commitment by the district. Any initial outlay should be recouped by improved practice with judicious use of time and increased satisfaction levels for both patients and staff. Making choices is inevitably a feature of health care whether at national level or at that of the individual but when finance is limited knowing that quality does not suffer is important.

Communications

Good communications are essential if an undertaking is to be successful. All staff should know what quality assurance means, because information clearly explained lessens stress and worry and of course gives people the opportunity early enough in an undertaking to question what is involved.

At the start of the programme and throughout its development publicize what is going on – talk to staff, perhaps send out a newsletter – not just a memo. Allow people to say what they feel about the innovation. If possible identify and allay their anxiety. Admit there may be grey areas and that you may not have all the answers for in most cases honesty and openness bring about trust. Give the staff opportunity to discuss what is happening, if necessary call meetings and at the meeting allow staff to talk through their feelings about the changes. Such meetings can be useful too for often others may identify something that has been missed or they may have better ideas on how to handle situations or identify priorities that are important in the clinical situation.

We mentioned that the plan should include the methodology to be used if it has been decided at this point. As this is such a crucial decision this question will now be considered in some depth.

The quality monitoring methodology

When considering the means by which quality is to be monitored and evaluated, there would seem to be three options:

1 Design an instrument specific to a particular department, unit or speciality, and determine its use.
2 Develop or modify an already established quality monitoring methodology.
3 Choose and use an already established quality monitoring methodology.

It is common to use the term 'instrument' to describe the means of measurement, we will refer to this in more detail in Chapter 3. It is a wise investment to carry out a literature search and to compile a bibliography and glossary of terms to ensure that the appropriate staff are given the chance to have access to the relevant information and the same understanding of the terminology to be used before any final decision is made. A particular help in this respect will be the Quality Assurance Information Service provided by the King's Fund in conjunction with the Department of Health library. Part of this service is to produce a bi-monthly abstract journal.

As implied earlier cost may be an important factor in deciding the first choice of methodology to be used or developed.

In choosing an already established methodology, consideration should also be given to one which has an accompanying patient dependency scale because this has the advantage of aiding managers in nurse manpower planning as well as having criteria that are applicable to certain dependency groups. However it has to be appreciated that this too must be introduced and tested with the same vigilance as the quality monitoring instrument itself. It should be said however that some adequate instruments do not have this facility but they should not be dismissed without considering what they have to offer.

Deciding on the monitoring procedure

Existing quality monitoring methodologies usually suggest the procedure to be used in monitoring quality. However now nurses are devising their own standards and criteria, the monitoring procedure part must be given much thought and effort. Those developing instruments should not be afraid to take advice and read what others are doing in this field, but a word of caution, do seek permission and acknowledge the work of others. The choice of what is to be monitored may well influence the time of day and the frequency. When devising the procedure look at what is realistic. Do you have the staff and finance to carry out monitoring more than three times a year? One also has to consider the processing of results, how is this to be done and by whom? How long will it take to send out the scores and to get a response from the charge nurse before monitoring quality again?

The selection of the target population of patients or the area to be monitored is of primary concern because this can influence the choice of methodology. There may be one available or one may need to be modified to suit a particular patient group. For example, in paediatric units, nurses could chose between Rush Medicus Quality Monitoring Methodology and the S.A.V.E. (selected attributes with variable evaluation) programme of the Sick Children's Hospital, Toronto (Jenkinson, 1981). There may not be reliably tested instruments available, for example for nursing in the community, although many are in different stages of development around the United Kingdom.

The results of consumer questionnaires and voluntary agency reports may be indicators for the choice and setting of standards and for the need to monitor specific topics. Consulting with other disciplines is important particularly if they are to be influenced by or can influence the quality scores. Hegyvary et al. (1979) found that the quality of nursing care is subject to considerable variations as a result of influences from non-clinical areas of the patient care systems.

If the results are to be scored manually by the person carrying out the monitoring do they have the skills to do this? It would seem sensible to make this as easy and as quick as possible – the scores should be easy to analyse and the means of presenting the results easy to do and to read. A computer would seem to be the answer; however they can be costly to buy, install and programme. Consideration must also be given to the training of the staff in the use of computers – with the increasing use of computers this would seem a wise investment for the future if funds are available.

Aids to evaluation

Many instruments do have an accompanying workbook – guidelines for the use of the methodology – and this is certainly a necessary adjunct to any quality monitoring methodology. For every new instrument a workbook should be produced. When monitoring, a manual of nursing procedures and policy statements applicable to the area being evaluated is useful. It is a wise investment to design some form of action plan (Table 2.2), which contains the scores and which will enable the ward, department, or community charge nurse to respond to the scores that may have been identified. Pocket calculators also have their uses.

Who monitors the quality?

Bergman (1982) posing the question of who should carry out the evaluation of nursing care, feels that employing an outside evaluator ensures greater objectivity, but warns that the report may have little use because of minimal involvement by local staff. It can however be argued that with a good educational programme objectivity can be maintained as effectively with local staff as with outsiders. Conversely staff can still respond to the findings of an outside evaluator if they are kept informed and findings presented in a positive manner.

Some units have a senior nurse and a charge nurse conducting the monitoring but not usually in their own ward – there are no hard or fast rules, it is something that has to be decided by the local steering group. The people carrying out the monitoring procedure may be called observers, raters, assessors, auditors or monitors. We have chosen the name observers.

The observers

The observers should be chosen for their ability to make professional and clinical judgements in a credible manner. They need to be able to anticipate and handle difficult situations should these arise, whilst at the same time maintaining a sensible and positive approach to evaluation. It should be remembered that even with the most reliable instrument there will always be a degree of subjective judgement. Therefore 'the observers, although guided by criteria and relevant information, have to listen and report accurately what they see and hear' (Kemp, 1986).

The education, practice and inter-observer reliability testing for the observer is crucial and should not be neglected. No one should be expected to carry out monitoring without having practised using the instrument and developed a sound knowledge of the methodology being used.

Within the education programme which will be discussed in Chapter 7 there will be inter-observer reliability testing. This means the level of agreement amongst observers, ie the percentage of time that two or more observers, collecting data from the same source at the same time, agree on what they have observed.

This is in fact a method of trying to ensure that the observers perceive the criteria similarly, thus aiding objective judgement. If the area of agreement is too low it may indicate that the criteria are not valid, or that the instrument is not reliable or valid for a particular area. It can also mean that the observers need further education and practice or, that through lack of experience or knowledge of the area to be evaluated, they are failing to understand what they are monitoring.

Practice in inter-observer reliability testing is also supportive of the observers, as it enables them to learn from each other and discuss any difficulties they may have. It should be carried out prior to the pilot study and repeated at least once a year if the instrument is to be accepted as reliable.

Preparation of staff

For people whose work or work area is to be evaluated this will involve being told about quality assurance and the purpose of the project. This should be done in a positive manner and not seen as a punitive exercise, and the reality of the situation should not be forgotten. People must know what exactly is expected of them and the implications of the programme. The quality monitoring methodology should be described and staff allowed to examine and discuss the instrument. It is important that all concerned staff are given time to discuss the proposals, to voice any fears they may have or difficulties they envisage. A method of reporting the progress of the innovations should also be planned. This is where the setting up of an educational backup programme is important as discussed in Chapter 7.

Setting up a pilot study

Whichever of the three options is chosen it is essential that the instrument be piloted and critically reviewed to ensure it suits the people and the environment involved. The choice of the area to be piloted should of course be a local decision and one fact that may influence the choice will be that the person responsible for the area is interested in and prepared to cooperate in having her work and that of the department evaluated. The charge nurse must be consulted and given as much information about the project as possible. A pilot study should not be imposed because it must be remembered that primarily the purpose of the pilot study is testing the reliability and validity of the instrument as well as the support system.

Review of the pilot study

After the pilot study has been completed it is necessary to critically look at the scores, the monitoring procedure and listen to the comments of the observers and those whose work was evaluated. It is a good idea to remind oneself of the purpose of the monitoring which was of course to pilot the quality monitoring methodology and critically review whether we have reached the objectives for the piloting. Did we give the correct education? Was enough time allowed for practice? Was enough regard given to the findings of the inter-observer reliability testing? Indeed, was it carried out at all? Were staff prepared? There is a need to look at the time factor and the cost involved, relook at the standards and criteria, some of them may need to be revised or discarded. This is hard work but a necessary task if a credible methodology is desired.

If you consider our flow chart (Table 2.1) you will see that if the piloting was satisfactory then you should go through the process of getting the standards ratified – meaning to receive approval and sanction, *Chambers Dictionary* (1980). This will obviously be sanctioned by the policy-making body of the unit. In the event that the instrument and monitoring procedure do not reach expectations then further work will need to be carried out on the weak areas. It would be very unfortunate and distressing for concerned staff if the whole quality monitoring system should need to be redesigned or a different instrument chosen, however, if this is needed, it must be done. It would of course reinforce the need for appropriate consultation and effective support systems to be used. Once the pilot study has been satisfactorily carried out and any modifications agreed, then the formal evaluation procedure will begin. This must follow consultation and discussion with the appropriate managerial and clinical staff. Individual methodologies will be discussed in more detail in later chapters.

Corrective action following routine monitoring procedure

The evaluation findings should be given as soon as possible after monitoring has been carried out, and the people who are to receive the findings should know when to expect them. The people who are going to receive the findings will obviously be the ward charge nurse or deputy or health visitor or a community charge nurse whose area of responsibility has been evaluated. The immediate managers will also get copies, for they are responsible for managing the service and supporting staff. The quality scores should also go to the manager of the unit to enable them to have an 'overview' of the level of care and performance.

Action plan

An action plan (Table 2.2) is provided for the charge nurse/team leader to respond in writing to the quality scores for their particular area of responsibility. It enables him/her to identify at a glance the strengths and weaknesses of their area, and to write down a plan to correct those weaknesses. It should not be seen as a punitive tool but rather a reinforcement of that which is good and a positive method of getting improvements made. It is also a record that the manager has been notified of the needs of the

Table 2.2 SUGGESTED QUALITY ASSURANCE ACTION PLAN

Ward, department, health centre

Quality assurance scores
To – Charge nurse/ward sister/community sister/community charge nurse/health visitors.
Response
(Please comment on scores, specifying the strengths and difficulties of the department, ward, non-institutional settings.)

Plan for corrective action

Priorities (set goals to improve scores that give cause for concern.)

Date for plan to be evaluated

Signature of charge nurse/sister/health visitor.
This form to be return to .... Please retain copy.

area. However these identified needs should be realistic and if they are not, the manager should explain, in writing, why they are not. If as a result of a second evaluation the scores have not improved, the needs of that area must be looked at seriously to see if the expectations are now too high or staff morale is low or that no action has been taken to improve performance by either the manager or the clinical staff. There is also the possibility that the instrument used is no longer reliable and valid for that area.

The development of quality assurance is in its early stages. It must be remembered that innovation necessitates behavioural changes which at times can be traumatic. It behoves us all to do our best to ensure these changes are carried out effectively.

Implementing change

Bringing in a quality assurance programme to an organization involves a change in the way that people are looking at and evaluating the work which they are doing and may subsequently modify and change their practices.

Any changes in organizational structure or activity may pose a threat to its members, and the NHS has certainly been exposed to an inordinate amount of change over the last 15–20 years.

Change has been described as a significant alteration in the status quo and is used here to mean an alteration which is beneficial to the people involved (Havelock, 1973). People within organizations will have different perceptions of the need for change depending on their place in the organization. Effective management of the situation therefore acknowledges this difference and makes sure that the correct information is given so that learning takes place at a pace which the individuals can handle and anxiety about change is kept to a minimum. It is also important to support and nurture the individuals through the change until the new pattern of behaviour is established. It is equally important to discover the reasons for resistance to change.

If clinical practitioners have had some involvement in developing or choosing a quality measuring instrument it will obviously have greater credibility with the users, and if they set the standards and criteria there will be an element of pride and, for most people, motivation to use the instrument.

The next chapter will look at what standards and criteria are, how to set them, and the question of their measurement.

References

Bergman R. (1982) Evaluation of nursing care – could it make a difference? *International Journal of Nursing Studies*. Vol 19, No 2. 53–60.

Macdonald A. M. ed. (1980) *Chambers Twentieth Century Dictionary*. Edinburgh: Chambers.

Chapman C. (1978) A philosophy of nursing practice and education. *Nursing Times*. February 23, 303–5.

Fitzgibbon M. (1986) Quality Assurance and Nursing Peer Review. Study Tour Report. Smith and Nephew, Florence Nightingale Scholarship. The Florence Nightingale Committee, London.

Griffin A. P. (1980) Philosophy and nursing. *Journal of Advanced Nursing*. **5**. 261–72.

Havelock R. (1973) *The Change Agents Guide to Innovation in Education*. New Jersey, USA: Educational Technology Publications Inc. Through Heath, *et al.* (1985) Introducing Change – Nursing Process in Practice. E.N.B. Resources Unit Sheffield.

Hegyvary S. T. (1979) Nursing process: the basis for evaluating the quality of nursing care. *International Nursing Review*. 26, **4**. 113–6.

Jenkinson V. (1981) *What is Quality Assurance?* King's Fund Project Paper. London: King's Fund Centre.

Kemp N. (1986) What is quality assurance? *The Professional Nurse*. February. Vol 1, 124–6.

King's Fund. *Quality Assurance Information Source*. London: King's Fund Centre.

McFarlane. Jean, Baroness Mcfarlane of Landaff (1982) Nursing values and nursing action. *Nursing Times*. September 29, 109–12.

Phelby D. F. H. (1982) Changing practice in confidentiality. A cause for concern. *Journal of Medical Ethics*. 8, **1**. 12–18.

Rush Medicus – Nursing Process Quality Monitoring Instrument. (1974) Public Health Service Contract No 1, Nu-24229. United States Department of Health, Education and Welfare. Washington D.C. 20402.

3

Standard setting

In this chapter we intend to focus on developing standards and criteria in an effort to help nurses devise means of measuring quality of care and performance. We expect readers will have their own reasons for setting standards which may include their motivation to enhance patient care and the means of clarifying what constitutes good practice.

Because of the complexity and the comparatively short experience of measuring quality of nursing care in the United Kingdom, we feel it would be helpful to the reader if we discussed five terms we will be using in this and the following chapters:

Instrument to measure quality, such an instrument enables nurses to measure the quality of nursing care; it can take the form of check lists, questionnaires or surveys. We see it as being composed of both standards and criteria, in a format that guides evaluation and enables a score of quality to be obtained. There are some quality instruments available that only contain standards, or only criteria which some people find satisfactory. Quality may also be measured by a panel of people auditing documentation (using the check-list type instrument) and/or discussing the results of care or performance. Some of these methods will be dealt with in greater detail later.

Evaluation for our purposes, means not only to judge the worth of something, but more specifically it is a means of finding out whether we have achieved what we set out to do when we planned care. We know from our experience that judgement involves elements of subjective and objective thought. Subjective involves assessments made from our feelings and attitudes, those things which are sometimes intangible. Objective involves things that can be observed and/or controlled 'uncoloured by one's own sensations' (*Chambers Dictionary*, 1980). It is because of these two sometimes conflicting elements that evaluation and thus measurement can be difficult, and it is for this reason that we need standards and criteria to guide and help us produce credible results. These we hope to explain as we go through this book. We also feel the following observation made by Bergman in 1982 may be of some help to nurses trying to understand the evaluation of nursing care. She believes 'that it is a combination of both the objective measurement of concrete phenomena, as well as subjective perceptions and opinions of the "feelings" of care as reported by recipients, providers and important others'.

Monitoring can be defined as checking care and performance with criteria against agreed standards to produce a measurement of quality. Monitoring, which enables evaluation to take place, is carried out by observers using an instrument that guides their observations and thus judgements.

This information can be obtained from one or a combination of the following sources:

- patient and nurse records
- patient and health carer interview
- observation of the patient, his/her care and environment
- observation of nursing practice and its management
- the provision of support services

Quality monitoring methodology is the method of measuring quality, or procedure, for evaluating care. It includes preparing the area and personnel for monitoring, using the instrument and processing the results.

Measurement, in its broadest sense is 'the assignment of numerals (or symbols) to objectives or events according to rules' (Stevens through Kitson, 1986). At its simplest it is the act of producing a score for some purpose. For quality to be evaluated in a satisfactory way, a scoring system should be used, because a numerical result more easily enables us to compare performance. It can also indicate that we should take action to correct deficiencies or to give praise, and enables choices to be made. The observations and responses noted by someone evaluating care are easier to deal with if they can be given a numerical value. A numerical score is also easier to produce if responses are only yes or no. With a numerical value, a percentage score for quality can be obtained. There is less chance of making an error of judgement when recording the observation of the presence or absence of factors than in instruments where the observer has to judge whether the criteria are demonstrating good or poor care; although some such statements do have a numerical value added to them to produce a numerical score for quality.

The development of standards and criteria

Standard is defined by *Chambers Dictionary* (1980) as 'a basis for measurement, an established or accepted model; a definite level of excellence or adequacy required, aimed at, or possible'. A working definition of standard which nurses may find useful is one given by the Royal College of Nursing; 'A standard is a professionally agreed level of performance appropriate to the population addressed, which is observable, achievable, measurable and desirable.' (RCN, 1986).

Example of a standard

The nursing process approach is the means of providing goal centred nursing care.

Criterion as defined by *Chambers Dictionary* (1980) is a 'means or standard of judging; a test; a rule'.

The Royal College of Nursing state that 'Criteria make standards work because criteria are detailed indicators of the standard and can be specific to the area or type of patient' (RCN, 1986).

For example, criteria for the above standard could include:

- Is there a written goal statement for each identified problem?
- Goals are evaluated on the date specified.

Criteria are in some instruments called interpretations, cues, characteristics or items. There would not seem to be any consensus of opinion as to what terms are the correct ones to use. This can be difficult for people trying to be precise and consistent. If you notice the two criteria written above, one is in the form of a question, one is a statement, however either one or the other can be used when writing criteria, as long as there is continuity and the observer knows what is required.

It seems that the word standard is generally accepted although some instruments do refer to their standard statements as objectives, sub-objective or items; whilst Mason (1984) uses a system which combines the standard and criterion in a single statement. Despite the confusion we will use the words standard and criteria – as does the Royal College of Nursing. When we are giving examples from the work of others, we will of necessity give the terms used in the work being shown. In simple words – standards are statements of intent and criteria are the means of measuring whether the standard has been reached or not.

Standards can originate in two ways:

1 'Normative standards derive, in principle, from the source that legitimately set the standards of knowledge and practice'
2 'Empirical standards are derived from actual practice' (Donabedian, 1966).

When setting standards, these two areas can cause conflict because of the difference between what is desirable and what is realistic, particularly at this time of scarce resources. This is without doubt a big area for debate because of the moral and political implications. For example is it right to set standards that staff and patients cannot reach when resources are not available? Should not standard setting demonstrate acceptable and desirable needs? If there is to be compromise it should not be at the expense of professional integrity.

There should surely not be any conflict about who sets the standards and criteria for patient care. These include people with knowledge and experience of the subject to be evaluated and of the policies/procedures and resources of the Unit.

Standards should be

Measurable – capable of expressing a result.
Realistic – meaning they can be achieved.
Appropriate – for the patient population to which it will be applied.
Desirable and Acceptable – for the above reasons and to ensure that

it does not offend against culture and professional ethics, policies or procedures.

Unambiguous – must have clear meaning, leaving no room for doubt; therefore we have to be careful of emotive terms or jargon and use the correct words.

Criteria statements should be

Related to the response one would expect for the particular standard being measured.

Descriptive of nursing responsibility or patient involvement, and/ or relevant resources.

Free of bias – 'each patient to whom a criterion is applied should have an equal opportunity to obtain a high score. For example skin condition for an aged patient and a youth might require different scales' (Zimmer, 1974).

Suitable for quantification and statistical treatment.

Be valid – this refers to the extent to which a criterion actually measures what it seeks to measure.

Reliable so as to provide data that is consistent and accurate, ie 'can be expected to produce the same score if repeated in the same situation, and the same score if different people use it in the same situation' (Barnett and Wainwright, 1987).

Whilst we are not suggesting that a local quality measuring instrument should be designed using research methods, we do feel that we must consider the above factors when developing the standards and criteria. For example, lack of validity may not be noticed until the instrument is tested, this is sometimes because nurses become so involved in developing the standard they do not notice that the criteria is not actually relevant to that particular standard.

With regard to unambiguous standards, as Mason (1984) points out 'some words such as: knows, understands, frequently, normal, and as possible, are open to a wide range of interpretations'. When setting standards and criteria nurses should scrutinize the words they use, to make sure they will be interpreted accurately.

We feel it relevant to mention criteria being statements of nurses responsibility. We do have to keep in mind that in some specialities there may be an overlap of responsibility and if standards are being written that involve the work of others, this will call for consultation, agreement and ideally a sharing of responsibility in the design of the standard and the action to be taken on the results.

An area of controversy concerning criteria development is whether different weights or values should be given to individual criteria or whether all criteria should have equal value; for the former, one requires time, money and the help of an expert with statistical skills. We feel that at this present time, local instruments should have criteria of equal value.

Some people write criteria as statements, as with standards, others in the form of questions or very briefly, for example

Standard: All newly qualified nurses receive education on Health and Safety at Work regulations

Criteria: Management Course
Tapes
Training manual

This method can be very worrying for the person who is going to carry out the evaluation or trying to understand what is being suggested. It is therefore a good idea when writing standards and criteria to ask the question – will the observers know what is required?

Jelinek et al. (1974) in discussing the development of the Rush Medicus Quality Monitoring Instrument, which was completed after much research and is now used by nurses in many countries, tells how 'to make criteria more consistent in terms of their likely interpretation by quality observers, they were frequently rewritten and expanded to give greater guidance to observers in their interpretation. The latter was achieved not only through identifying the source of information by which the specific evaluation was to be made, but also by providing follow-on probe questions that would tend to elicit extra relevant information.' It is interesting to note that they too had to rewrite some of their work, we should not get disheartened when we have to do the same. Of particular interest is the guidance to the observers, because it seems to us that many people are devising standards and criteria without any guidance on what questions need to be asked or observations made to ensure the instrument is used correctly. We also have to remember that if we are not careful we may be manipulating the responses people make by leaving each observer to devise his/her own questions, which in turn may influence the reliability of the instrument.

You will find an example of material taken from the Rush Medicus Quality Monitoring Instrument to illustrate the previous points:

DATA

SOURCE

Sub-Objective (read standard)

THE PATIENT IS PROTECTED FROM ACCIDENT AND INJURY.

CRITERION. Are safety measures, such as smoking regulations or precautions, getting in and out of bed, explained on admission to the unit. Code not applicable if patient admitted to another unit (ward).

PATIENT

INTERVIEW

ASK PATIENT: When you arrived on this unit (ward) were you told if there was some special safety measures on this unit, such as smoking regulations or precautions getting in or out of bed, or any other precautions.

TO GIVE ORDER TO STANDARD SETTING

Donabedian's (1969) approach to evaluation of quality is a useful guide, because it reminds us of the different domains involved in health care. These are structure, process and outcome. *Structure* refers to factors in the organization that enables work to be carried out; such as environmental facilities, equipment, staffing, educational facilities, personnel and management.
Process refers to the performance – the care the health provider gives to the patient and or the community.
Outcome is the end result of care and performance, the effect of care on the patient, people significant to him and the community.

It is relevant that we make some comment about these factors, which we will develop in the following chapters. With regard to *structure*, one cannot look at the quality of nursing care in totality without having a view of those things that aid nursing care.

'It is thought by some that because *process* focuses on what the health carer does it should be easier to measure, however how does one measure those aspects of care that come from the nurse's experience, sensitivity and empathy for the patient and his family?' Kemp (1984). These are not easy to measure however they have to be considered if we are going to evaluate the process of care.

Outcome can be seen as the most worthwhile of all the measures, trying to ensure that what we planned and carried out was worthwhile and effective. Yet again a word of caution has to be given. This is not easy, it is probably the most difficult area to evaluate effectively, because of the complexity of nursing, the multifactorial input to care and all the intangible things that influence the patient and what he feels about his care.

There is also debate whether one can truly evaluate practice and performance using only one of these three domains, or should all aspects of the three be included. It is possible to set standards for structure, for process and for outcome combining all three into one instrument and using the relevant criteria. It is also possible to devise an instrument using standards in only one of the domains. The thing to remember is that we are all at this time breaking new ground and there are no hard and fast rules about which domain to use. It very much depends on what the instrument is needed for. The nurses of West Berkshire Health Authority (Kendall 1987) use a method whereby they write a general standard statement with criteria based on structure, process and outcome as shown in Table 3.1.

Preparation for and procedure to develop a quality measuring instrument

The group that sets the standards and criteria may be at regional, district, unit level, or within specialities. We have decided to focus on nurses setting standards and developing a quality monitoring methodology for direct patient care at ward/department level within a speciality or within a team of community nurses. The same principles of consultation, discussion and effective communications, as discussed in Chapter 2, applies just as much to the smaller group as to the unit or district wide group. It is likely that most standard setting groups within a district will have some connection to a group at unit or district level, for example the district group may have the duty of ratifying the

Table 3.1   TABLE 3.1 IS A DRAFT COPY OF A STANDARD AND CRITERIA THAT WAS USED BY NURSES WORKING IN GROUPS ON MONITORING STANDARDS AND WAS DEVISED BY HELEN KENDALL WHILST WORKING FOR WEST BERKSHIRE HEALTH AUTHORITY.

WEST BERKSHIRE HEALTH AUTHORITY

STANDARD REFERENCE NO. _____

TOPIC: __CONTINUITY__

SUB-TOPIC: __DISCHARGE PLANNING__

CARE GROUP: __HOSPITAL PATIENTS__

ACHIEVE STANDARD BY: _____

REVIEW STANDARD BY: _____

THIS STANDARD IS APPLICABLE IN THE FOLLOWING WARDS/DEPARTMENTS/AREAS: _____

SIGNATURE OF D.N.S. _____

SIGNATURE OF SENIOR NURSE _____

DATE _____

STANDARD STATEMENT: Each patient's discharge from hospital is planned and carried out in accordance with his needs, abilities and wishes.

STRUCTURE	PROCESS	OUTCOME
The nurse has local knowledge of services available.	The nurse includes in the Nursing Record: Assessment of factors affecting discharge, the views of patient and relative, home circumstances, where relevant.	A discharge plan is completed for each patient.
Reference: Resource book of services available in each ward.		The support services detailed in the plan are arranged.
The nurse knows how to contact the Senior Nurse, Community Liaison for advice; and the patient's District Nurse for exchange of information.	The nurse plans preparation for discharge and sets goals for discharge with patient and relative.	The patient's discharge and aftercare is in accordance with his individual needs and wishes.
	The nurse coordinates arrangements for transfer and the support services required.	The patient and/or relative achieve the discharge goals.
The policy for discharge arrangements W.B.H.A.: Transfer of patients from hospital to Community No. 1 is available in the ward.		The patient and/or relative can explain the discharge instructions.
	The nurse provides teaching time and written instructions for each patient and/or relative before discharge.	No complaints related to discharge or transfer arrangements.
A Nursing History form, which includes the details of family and home circumstances and a format for discharge planning, is available for each patient.	The nurse evaluates the pre-discharge teaching.	

Reproduced by permission of Helen Kendall

H. Kendall.

quality measuring instrument which has been developed at local level.

There are advantages of local staff developing their own standards and quality measuring instrument. The instrument thus developed will be based on local needs and professional knowledge. It will provide a sense of pride and be owned by the group. However it would be remiss of us if we did not point out that there is much duplication of effort throughout the United Kingdom. Should we not perhaps be questioning whether this is an appropriate use of scarce resources?

The RCN have developed the Dynamic Standard Setting System (Kitson, 1988), based on the work at West Berkshire. This system 'involves groups of ward staff setting standards, monitoring and evaluating their own practice. It takes a problem solving approach, where topics for quality improvement are identified by the group, criteria formulated, a standard statement agreed and measurement techniques determined. The final

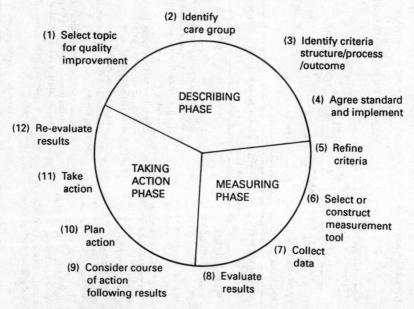

Fig. 3.1 The Quality Assurance Cycle

The RCN dynamic standard setting approach: the Q.A. cycle. Reproduced with permission of Alison Kitson

part involves the group in agreeing appropriate courses of action which are subsequently evaluated in the light of the agreed standards.' This is illustrated in the diagram based on Lang's model by Kitson (Fig. 3.1).

This system does presume a quality assurance advisory committee at district/area level, and a quality assurance coordinating committee which represents functional units of patient care management either geographically or by speciality. The work of the Quality Assurance Standard Setting teams would take place at a functional level. Kitson (1988) points out 'the system is decentralized at ward/unit level. However it is coordinated in a manner that ensures standards of care travels across each of the units within the district/area board.' If this kind of organization could be implemented throughout districts – communications would be enhanced and the work of nurses trying to implement quality assurance systems would be made easier.

We would make the point that whilst this dynamic system is a very useful guide and could be of great benefit to all health professionals. We feel that the model suggests that criteria are developed before the standard is considered, in fact because the topic has been chosen the standard is given some thought but not refined until the criteria have been devised and discussed. We prefer the method of developing the standard before selecting the criteria, however it is the method that the group decides suits them best that matters!

Composition of the group

The group setting the standards should not be too large, certainly not more than six persons and ideally not less than four. It is our experience that over six is too unwieldy. Less than four means that too much work has to be carried out by the members and often the group becomes 'too cosy' and not enough discussion or healthy disagreement takes place. It is a good idea to have a cross section of nurses from the clinical area and, when possible, a clinical teacher or tutor within the group because these different grades of people bring different perspectives to the work particularly as it relates to the views and needs of patients.

It is obviously sensible to have the backing of the senior manager for local initiatives, for not only will they be in a position to provide support and reasonable resources. They may also fulfil the role of *coordinator*. This person could 'coordinate, monitor and evaluate all standards setting initiatives within her/his clinical area of responsibility' (Portsmouth and South East Hampshire Health Authority, 1988).

People with particular responsibility in the group are the: *Group Leader* – ideally a charge nurse/sister. She or he will be responsible for selecting the team, arranging and conducting the meetings and reporting on the work to the manager/coordinator.

Of great help to a group would be a *Facilitator*. This enabling role should be taken by someone with knowledge of quality assurance, teaching and group dynamics – perhaps the nurse teacher or a nurse with some research experience because this person's task is to help without dictating and to support the group leader when necessary. Some health districts do provide facilitators to help with their quality initiatives. However many groups are having to get on with the job without such help.

Individual roles of people within the group should be clarified and the responsibility and authority for specific role function should be made clear. Ideally this should be planned by the clinical nurse who is going to be group leader and the manager. It will also be useful if simple role descriptions are written, because they do help group members to feel secure and tends to keep them 'on the right path'.

The group should meet at least twice a month otherwise the members may loose their momentum. The time the group takes at each meeting is a matter of preference but not less than one hour or more than two would seem sensible. However only experience will tell what is best for a particular group. The place a group meets should also be given some thought, a place that is comfortable and free of interruption is to be preferred.

The work of the group follows in principle the framework we described in Chapter 2 (Table 2.1). The first task for the group members should be to examine and write out its purpose, develop a philosophy, choose or devise a definition of quality, and draw up a plan with objectives. A decision should be made as to what facilities are required and if they are available, for example, are particular resource people available and can they be consulted and or employed?

It is sensible to carry out a literature search, compile a glossary and examine the relevant research for the speciality, all of which could help with standard setting. It is a good idea to check if anyone else in the district is doing similar work, because they may already have some of this information which they would be willing to share. The RCN professional groups may also have information that could be helpful. If necessary write some simple guidelines for the group members.

In developing a philosophy it is very important that the group discuss what standard setting means to them. It cannot be presumed that all the members will have the same values, commitment or motivation towards standard setting. It is a good idea for the person leading this discussion to consider what the standards will mean to the patient, those significant to him, and the unit in which the nurses work, the nursing profession and society. If effective work is to be achieved, this situation has to be discussed and any problems confronted with honesty and sensitivity.

It is important that the group produces or chooses a working definition of quality, this should be easier if the group has looked at its philosophy and values. Some people might feel it is impossible to define quality and thus time wasting, but discussing what quality means enables nurses to clarify their thoughts on the subject and may identify further needs. The definition will act as a guideline not only to the group but to others interested in the work.

At this point educational input may be beneficial. Members of the group may need to know what standards and criteria are, they may need to be able to practise devising both, in an atmosphere that is conducive to experiential learning. There should be time to think, criticise and to praise. It may be a good idea to ensure that any group undertaking standard setting be reminded of how groups work. Above all things the group members should be allowed time to talk and identify fears, difficulties and strengths; this is where a skilled facilitator could prove very useful.

Whilst we have tried to put the above steps in order, in practice they may be implemented differently.

Choosing the topics to be evaluated

First choose the patient group, this may be homogeneous in that the standards will be expected to relate equally to all the patients and staff within that speciality or a specific group which may be identified by age, gender, diagnosis, disease or discipline.

The topic or topics to be selected may be chosen because they are giving cause for concern – such as poor communications or it may be an innovation that wants evaluating. It should be remembered that evaluative mechanisms should be designed not only to be used to identify deficiencies but also to re-inforce good practices and good outcomes.

We feel that if standards are to be set for more than one topic or area the use of some kind of framework is of help because it acts as a reminder of what is planned and sometimes why. This may be based on a needs approach or a model relevant to the speciality. The group may develop its own framework. Whichever is chosen, consider drawing it or writing it out. For example the following framework was used in a project that set standards of care for people resident in long-term care (Fig. 3.2).

Selecting the format of the instrument

After deciding the topics to be evaluated, consider in which domain, ie structure, process and or outcome, the standards and criteria are to be developed. We feel, although not everyone would agree, that before starting to set the standards there is a need to decide on the format of the instrument and decide how the standards are to be measured. It is quite useful to look at established instruments for ideas, bearing in mind that some are stored on computer and therefore the acutal sheet on which to note the scores may be separated from the standards and criteria.

The format that was developed by Helen Kendall and the nurses in West Berkshire Health Authority, shown on page 37, does presume a nurse management structure that is able to ratify standards, and does seem to indicate that each standard is to be checked by a senior nurse and the director of nursing–this would seem to be a vast undertaking, always supposing the two nurses have the time alongside their other responsibilities. However in answer to this observation Kendall (1989, personal correspondence) points out 'each senior nurse manager is responsible for maintaining/monitoring standards of care in their units.' She feels agreement of standards is not an arduous

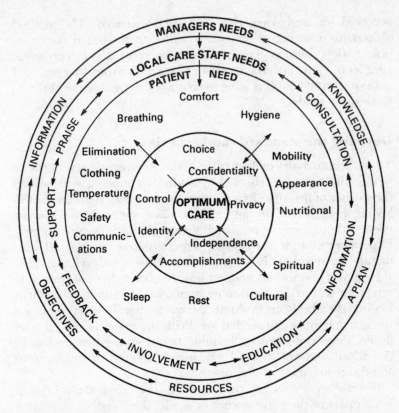

Fig. 3.2 The framework is based on a needs approach: From the periphery the two outer circles indicate the needs of the managers, and local care staff, to enable them to support the undertaking. Moving inwards we come to two further circles. The outer of which contains the topics on which the standards and criteria are based – however every time a standard is set the question should be asked, have the intangible issues, which are highlighted in the inner circle, been considered? The nucleus of the framework, is the goal of optimum care.

Source: Kemp and Sander. Unpublished Work, 1988.

task when it is related to a senior nurse's specific area of expertise. With this format there is no indication on how the standards are to be measured and where the scores are to be noted. However, there is a reminder when the standards are to be achieved by, and when they are to be reviewed. The method of making a standard statement with criteria based on structure, process and outcome would also seem a common sense approach. If the criteria are set out, one under the other it would save space and enable a score to be placed along side the observations to be made.

Devising the standards and criteria

There are no hard or fast rules about how many standards to write. The topic for which the standards are being written and their order of priority often dictates the number. We offer the following suggestions; do not have too many for each component/need, although one is not usually enough, initially aim for two. Experience and the needs of the target group of patient will often dictate the number. If too many standards are developed, consider getting statistical help on how to divide them up into subsets, that will make them more manageable without necessarily loosing the ability to evaluate a cross section of the population the instrument was intended for. With the easier access to computers there is now more flexiblity because programmes can be developed that only use subsets, ie only a certain number of the standards are used at any one time.

To commence setting the standards the group should decide which part of their framework or model they wish to start with. A group may choose a topic that seems the easiest to start with – because it is very reassuring to have some success at the start of a project. The group may choose one of the following options:

1   Each member of the group writes one standard.
2   The group discusses what the standard should be and one person writes down what is decided.
3   The members use a 'brain storming technique' to decide what should be in the standard, with one member writing down the ideas.

Whichever option is used the group members should together kindly critique what has been done, this should be followed either by selecting and refining or rejecting the work or just choosing the standard and going straight on to develop the criteria coming back to refining or rejecting the standard in the light of the experience of developing the criteria.

With criteria development decide what is needed for that particular standard, discuss local practices and look for new acceptable ideas, and at the research for that subject. One can use the options 2 and 3 as above for criteria development. If discussing some specialist element of care try to get help from the specialist, for example, a Nutritional Nurse Adviser. Do remember that, as with standards, criteria must be professionally acceptable. When deciding which criteria to use, we must remember that some are mandatory, for example, those that relate to safety. One cannot alter the policies of a Health Authority to suit that instrument development. However the result of using the instrument may show that policies need updating.

It is a good idea, from time to time, to look critically at what is being achieved by the group, check the standards and criteria: do they make sense – try reading them out loud, are they ambiguous? Would an observer know what questions to ask or observation to make? Do the standards and the criteria seem measurable? Does the standard and the criterion both have the characteristics necessary to be effective. Group members should be careful they do not introduce bias by allowing their own prejudices to creep into the wording of the standard statement – for example 'All patients shall be clean and tidy.' This seemingly innocent statement may not suit the philosophy of some nurses and more importantly some patients.

In ideal circumstances nurses would involve patients in standard setting; for without doubt this is of benefit to the patient and the nurse. The patient will often identify priorities and needs that are important to him, which the nurse may not have thought about. This may then be brought to the group for consideration. When one of the authors did this a patient said 'I know I stink, I sweat a lot and most of the time I find I can't stand me – so it must be awful for everybody else – could you do something about it? – so people like me aren't an embarrassment to others and ourselves.' The standard was written which the nurse and the patient looked at together, they then planned the criteria, and together, they evaluated the worthiness of what they had written. Which is as follows:

Standard

Help is given discreetly to patients to enable them to cope with
    potentially embarrassing hygiene problems

Criterion (only one example noted here)

A patient who is uncomfortable or socially isolated because of excessive perspiration is discreetly offered, talcum powder, anti-perspirant, or deodorant (unless contra-indicated).

Instruction to observer: If the problem is identified or odour is obvious but no action plan is written code 'no'. If a plan of action is written which meets the criteria code 'yes'.

The above standard was developed by Nattrass, Kemp and Sander, for the project 'Quality of life in long-stay care.' Wessex Regional Health Authority, (1988) unpublished work.

Remember that we indicated earlier that standards and criteria may need to be written and refined many times.

Having devised the standards and criteria and selected the format for the instrument, consider the way the instrument is to be used and the way in which the scores are going to be presented. Then set about testing the instrument. In an ideal world there would be money to have it tested by a research team. If not, pilot the instrument using the guidelines as discussed in Chapter 2, making sure the nurses carrying out the pilot study know the requirements for a standard and criterion. It is worthwhile even with a small instrument to carry out inter-observer reliability testing which can be defined as the level of agreement among observers. Reliability refers to the repeatability of observation (ie, what percentage of the time two or more observers collecting data from the same source at the same time agree on what they observe) cited by Kemp (1983). Standards and criteria can be validated by a panel of experts, however we think there is no substitute for testing an instrument in the area in which it is planned to use it.

Having tested the instrument, and consulted concerned people and reviewed the methodology – send it to the policy making body to be ratified. A decision should be made as to when an instrument is to be reviewed, techniques and sometimes philosophies change, therefore any quality monitoring methodology should be kept up-to-date.

We feel it would not be right if we ended this chapter without a further word on measurement and the level at which quality can be set. Many people are trying to set standards without confronting the issue of how their standards are to be measured, and how scores will be produced and presented, unfortunately little is written that is easily understood; therefore, if in doubt, keep the scoring simple. If funds are available, employ a statistician. With regard to the level of quality, people are using such terms as: minimum, optimum and maximum which sound very good but unless these terms are defined and assigned a numerical value they are meaningless in measurement terms.

Without doubt developing an instrument to measure the quality of nursing care is a big undertaking and it is not easy, however it is enabling nurses to demonstrate their commitment to patients, the community, colleagues and the nursing profession. It is a chance to influence and perhaps change society for the good of all people. We must not miss this opportunity.

References

Barnett D., Wainwright P. (1987) Between two tools. *Senior Nurse*. vol. 6, no 4. April. 40–42.

Bergman R. C. (1982) Evaluation of Nursing Care – could it make a difference? *International Journal of Nursing Studies*. vol. 19 no 2 53–60

Macdonald A. M. ed (1980). *Chambers Twentieth Century Dictionary*, Edinburgh: Chambers.

Donabedian A. (1966) Evaluating the quality of medical care. Millbank Memorial Fund. Quarterly vol. 44 166–203.

Donabedian A. (1969) Some issues in evaluating the quality of nursing care. *American Journal of Public Health*. vol. 59. no 10. 1833–6.

Jelinek R. C., Haussmann R. K. D., Hegyvary S. T. and Newmann T. F. A Methodology for Monitoring Quality of Nursing Care. U.S. Department of Health Education and Welfare. DHEW Publication No (HRA) 74–25 January 1974, Washington D.C. 20402: U.S. Government Printing Office.

Kemp N. 1983. Quality Assurance and the Nursing Process. Florence Nightingale/Smith and Nephew Scholarship, Report. p. 56. London: The Florence Nightingale Committee.

Kemp N. (1984) A place for quality. *Senior Nurse*. vol. 1, no 34. November 12–16.

Kendall H. (1987) Royal College of Nursing – Workshop for Nurse Managers on setting standards. 14 April. London: Royal College of Nursing.

Kitson A. (1986) Quality Assurance – The method of measuring quality. *Nursing Times*. August 27. 32–4.

Kitson A. (1988) Nursing Quality Assurance – Dynamic standard setting system. RCN Standards of Care project. 11 February. London: The Royal College of Nursing.

Mason E. J. *How to Write Meaningful Standards. (1984)*. 2nd ed. New

York: J. Wiley & Sons, Medical Publication.

Portsmouth and South East Hampshire Health Authority. Nursing and Midwifery Advisory Standard Setting Group. (1988) Portsmouth, England.

RCN 1986. Standards of care project. Check list on how to write standards of nursing care. 16 December. London: Royal College of Nursing.

Rush Medicus – Nursing process quality monitoring instrument. (1974) Public Health Service Contract No 1, Nu – 24299. January. Washington D.C. 20402. United States Department of Health, Education and Welfare.

Zimmer M. J. (1974) Guidelines for development of outcome criteria. *Nursing Clinics of North America*. vol. 9. no 2. June. 2317–21.

4

The caring environment and quality

In setting out to evaluate the quality of the environment it is useful to have determined a particular approach as we indicated in Chapter 3. Donabedian (1969) suggests that 'one may classify these approaches under three headings: structure, process and outcome'. When he talks about 'structure' he is referring to the environment in which care is given.

As his categories are so universally known we have decided to use these three headings to discuss the evaluation of quality in this and the next two chapters. It can be argued that no one category is more important than the other. In some quality monitoring instruments elements of structure, process, and outcome standards are included. In order to give some framework to our thinking about standard setting we have chosen to separate and develop them in isolation. However, we must remember as Regis McKenzie (1979) writing in the *Lamp* states 'The structural component of quality assurance is as essential as the process and outcome components. All three elements are essential if a system is to be developed. One must complement the other, without one the others are not possible.' We hope that by reading this book the reader will have an appreciation of this statement.

We have said that when we talk about the domain of structure we are referring to the environment in which care is being given, we must now be rather more specific in what we mean by this. It may be reasonable to start by looking at Donabedian's (1969) own definition of structure.

The evaluation of structure consists in the appraisal of the instrumentalities of care and of their organization. It includes the properties of facilities, equipment, manpower and financing. It is the major approach used in drawing specifications for assessment, certification or accreditation. It assumes that when certain specified conditions are satisfied good care is likely to follow.

We are not yet used in the UK to processes of accreditation of our health care agencies but we are certainly familiar with the need to look at equipment, manpower, and financing in respect of care. It is interesting too to read the last sentence which makes the assumption that the satisfaction of specified conditions is likely to be followed by good care. There is a need for caution here and we must remind ourselves again of the very important integration of process and outcome along with structure. This is echoed by E. A. Will (1983) writing about quality assurance in *Nursing in the New Zealand Hospital* when she says that

> An evaluation of structure examines the setting in which care is given and includes assessment of the facility, equipment, supplies, manpower, support services and finance. It is necessary to ensure resources are available but if used in isolation is no guarantee of excellence of care.

In this statement there is commitment to look at the whole organization concerned with the provision of health care. Each part of the organization has specific areas of concern. Those who provide support services are attempting to evaluate the quality of the work they do, the same applies to medical provision and to the work of the paramedical staff. Together they combine to fulfil the purpose or mission of the organization and do so at a level by which quality is assured.

We are concerned with the part nursing plays in this and evaluating the structure in which nursing care is given. We will be looking in this chapter then at the setting of standards which relate to manpower, resources and facilities available.

Manpower

The purpose of a manpower planning system is to ensure that resources are used effectively. This means, among other things, that the 'right' number and grade of staff are allocated to each area where care is being given. One of our considerations is to look at what is meant by the 'right' number and grade of staff.

Historically the determination of nurse staffing levels has been based on tradition. No well tested methods were used. In fact it has been suggested that 'she who shouted loudest got the largest slice of the cake'. Was this management by screaming? This was reflected in the 'feast and famine' situation that many are familiar with but it does suggest that the determination of staffing levels was often based on emotional demands rather than on empirical evidence. They were certainly not linked initially to standards of nursing practice.

A study by the National League of Nursing Education (1937) in the hospitals of New York city attempted to equate staffing levels to hours of bedside nursing care and came up with a figure of 3.5 hours per patient per day. It was acknowledged at the time that this figure was a recommendation based on what appeared to be right for that time and that there was a need for further study. However, 30 years later a survey of hospitals in Canada (Canadian Nurses Association, 1966) revealed that this figure was still being used to estimate numbers of nursing staff.

Gionavetti (1979) cites that it was in the 1950s when studies began to suggest that the number of nurses needed should be based on the intensities of nursing care required rather than on the medical diagnosis. Of particular interest perhaps is the George and Kuehn (1955) study which indicated that there was a need to consider the health education needs of the mildly ill and the emotional reactions of the moderately ill as factors determining the types and intensities of nursing care and the time required.

In the following decade, work done at the John Hopkins Hospital (Connor, 1960) and elsewhere for the first time showed 'quantitatively' – that some patients need more care than others. In particular they showed that nursing workload depended on the number of patients in each category of care present on the ward. Two other findings of significance were that nursing workload varied from day to day and shift to shift and that wards differed. The last important criteria being that the main factor determining total nursing workload was the number of patients requiring intensive nursing care.

Since this time there has been a proliferation of studies both in North America and Britain so that now there is available a number of classification systems of patient dependency and staffing methods. Most of these schemes have at some time had their validity and reliability criticized. Definitions abound and terms are often used interchangeably.

The problem has to some extent been made worse by the fact

that there are no nationally or even regionally laid down standards for manpower planning. Many systems are available; some health authorities have used these directly or modified them for their own use, while still others have designed their own system to meet their particular needs.

In the North West Region a system was developed known as Criteria for Care – the manual of the North West Staffing Levels Project. The system 'consists of two major aspects; the first is the collection of data on workload, nursing activity and the level of patient care being achieved; the second is the formation of an information matrix upon which decisions about the most effective deployment of staff, and the optimum levels of staff required to deliver a high standard of care can be based' (Ball et al., 1984). The quality aspect of care is recorded by using Index for Care – Monitor, which will be discussed in Chapter 5.

The use of a patient dependency categorization system could be built into the standards set by a health authority. This may be at a number of different levels as for instance those written as regional standards for Wessex. In their recently published document (March, 1989) Standards for Nursing Services in the Wessex Region, standard 3 states:–

> Nurses shall use a valid patient dependency assessment system on a continuous basis to determine the numbers, grades and skill mix of nursing staff required to meet patient needs for nursing care. Any variations between the numbers of nurses needed by grades and skills and the actual numbers deployed shall be reported regularly to management.

A number of criteria relating to this standard have then been established. These include:–

> The systems used to measure patient dependency are:
> Applied to nursing services in all units/specialities
> Approved for use by the district nursing adviser
>
> The report to management on the variations between the results of the patient dependency assessment system and actual nurse deployment includes reference to the number of hours spent by nurses on non-nursing duties; and recommendations for changes designed to improve nurses effectiveness and/or efficiency

One other quite different source of information about nursing manpower lies in the Government-produced performance indicators. These indicators first published by the DHSS in

1983 cover a wide range of factors which one would expect to find as the core activities of any health district. They were produced 'to help those responsible for the delivery of health services. . . run their services more effectively'. They are in fact ratios which are based on centrally held statistical information collected from regions. This information has been gathered in an attempt to look at measures which contribute to quality of care. A district's relative performance in relation to other districts on any one indicator can raise questions which need to be explored. Many district health authorities at this present time have used them to consider services provided to individual client groups.

A consideration of a particular indicator illustrates their relationship to staffing levels. From the Performance Indicator package we can extract information about health visitor staffing which will tell us e.g. the number of health visitors per 1000 under 5-year-old children. It will also give the contact rate for health visitors with the over 65-year-olds. Further indicators will give the numbers of qualified health visitors which can be set against the number of unqualified staff working with them.

From the information which indicators like this can give standards can be set. In the case quoted above the standard would relate to provision of health visitor care and would be determined locally in agreement with local staff.

In nursing some of our staffing standards in areas where student nurses gain clinical experience are determined by criteria laid down by the National Boards. In the documents produced by the boards referred to as 'Institutional and Course Approval/Re-approval Process' there are included references to criteria for practical placements.

The standard statement with respect to practical placements is 'The quality of care and facilities provided for clients/patients must be such as to provide optimum learning to take place'. The specific criteria relating to manpower in this context is 'A minimum of one appropriately qualified first level nurse must be available, in a ward or department, to supervise students on each shift.'

Schools of nursing are in any case also required to audit their learning areas at least annually. The National Boards guidelines then may be used, or adapted, by the schools in setting their own criteria.

We have seen above that the supervision of student nurses

is the responsibility of an 'appropriately qualified first level nurse' and this statement leads us into a consideration of the 'appropriateness' of qualifications as part of structure standards. If quality is to be upheld then it is not enough to have sufficient manpower to staff the wards and departments of our hospitals but that manpower must be at a level which is agreed professionally as capable of providing good care. This is perhaps a particularly pertinent point at this time when we are considering the introduction of a new worker into the health service, namely the Health Care Assistant. If he/she is to be a support to the qualified nurse then we must be sure that we know what qualifications he/she needs and what preparation he/she will need to practice.

In Britain it is often a requirement that a nurse working in a specialist unit should hold the specialist qualification appropriate to that unit before appointment, or be willing to acquire that qualification as soon as is practical after appointment. Referring again to the National Board's approval document the criteria for a learning environment does include the statement:– 'The trained staff should, where appropriate, hold the qualification which is relevant to the particular care area.'

The registration of nurses in this country, and thus their licence to practise is laid down by act of Parliament. The latest legislation being contained within the Nurses, Midwives and Health Visitors Act of 1979. Registration being necessary to protect a vulnerable public from the vagaries of unauthorized practitioners.

The Act quite clearly lays down the standard required of someone who wishes to have her name on the Register and therefore be authorized to practise. Section 11(2) states that 'the applicant shall be registered. . . if she satisfies the Council that she is of good character and has the appropriate professional qualifications'. The Act then goes on to specify what it regards as 'the appropriate professional qualifications'. The quality of the staff providing care is surely the most important resource element we have but there are others.

Resources and facilities

Let us now turn our attention to other forms of resource within the environment in which care is given. A source of information on the provision of environmental facilities are consumer surveys. These may be done at national level by bodies such as the College of Health as referred to in Chapter 1; but they are also done at both regional and district level where they may be used directly to set standards for the provision of such facilities.

At local level it is quite often groups like the Community Health Councils who initiate such studies as part of their remit to act on behalf of the local consumers of health care.

One such survey was carried out by the Community Health Council in Salisbury. It was concerned to look at the local out-patient clinics and had three objectives. These were defined as:

1 To assess the impact of the out-patients department as the 'shop window' of the Salisbury Health Authority.
2 To investigate the effectiveness of the appointment procedure.
3 To ascertain the satisfaction of the consumer with the quality of service received.

Under the first objective a whole range of environmental factors were examined including the heating, lighting and ventilation of the out-patients hall itself. It also included a consideration of amenities such as provision of refreshments. The second objective was quite specific and examined the times of waiting in relation to both receiving appointments and the waiting subsequent to arrival at the hospital. Although the survey indicated a high degree of satisfaction in the quality of the service which was provided, several areas were identified as requiring attention in order to improve this. These areas were concerned with communications and attitudes in the main.

As a result of this survey the district agreed to produce a set of standards for the department 'to ensure that patients are offered a high quality service'. These standards determine amongst other things, the environment which should be provided for patients coming into out-patients.

They include–

Desks will be located where they can be easily seen and will display signs giving clear instructions to patients.

The location of vending machines for beverages and snacks, hospital shops and canteens will be clearly signposted. Toilets will be clearly signposted.

These standards have been agreed and are now being used to monitor the quality of care in the environment.

The support services in health care areas work together with nurses to ensure that the provision of environmental services are of a standard which will ensure quality. The East Dorset Health Authority have also examined the service provided to out-patients and have included standards which apply to other disciplines.

As an example a standard for the pharmacy department is

Patients who are prescribed items from the pharmacy at their out-patient appointment can obtain those items without any undue delay.

and for medical records is

Up-to-date medical records are always readily available in advance of the out-patient appointment.

included in the criteria set against that particular standard are

1 A record of all out-patient appointments is made in the patient's case notes;
2 The results of tests arranged by a general practitioner, prior to the out-patient appointment, are included in the case notes;
3 There are clear, agreed arrangements for patients referred to the out-patient department from casualty department at all times;

These give some indication of the range of structure standards which can be used within one hospital department.

A second source of information which may enable structure standards to be formulated may be the work done by Quality Circles. Quality Circles were first developed and used widely in Japan after the Second World War where they were found mainly in high-tech industries (Orlikoff and Snow, 1984). It was in these settings that they were first used when the idea was introduced in the United States in the mid 70s, but later were used more widely including in service industries.

They can be described very briefly as:—

'A group of five to eight people from the same work area that meet regularly to solve work-related problems.'

These problems may be related to a number of issues but quite frequently do throw up difficulties which are related to resources such as fittings and fixtures and to other forms of equipment.

In this country the work of quality circles set up in the North Warwickshire Health Authority is interesting. Their definition of quality circles throws more light on the work of such groups.

> They are a process in which every layer of an organization works together as a team to improve the quality of production, products, services and work life. (Hyde, 1984 Ed.)

An elaboration on this statement suggests that they are also a means of improving communication within the organization and enabling people to have greater involvement in improving patient care, and thus to have greater job satisfaction.

Quoted examples of the improvements which have been made as a result of the work of quality circles include an investigation into the number of accidents occurring in the ward. As a result of this work an identified cause of the accidents was found to be the hold handles in the toilet areas. A change in equipment and practices associated reduced the number of accidents. The findings of quality circles may be used to write standards which incorporate the improved practices.

Other circumstances may give rise to the need to write standards. Patient safety is a very important part of caring. Standards related to this have been produced by nurses at Salisbury. e.g.

Standard
Staff and equipment will be adequately prepared to cope with emergencies.

some of the related criteria are

Criteria
1 All nursing staff will attend a fire lecture/demonstration twice a year
2 All fire exits will be kept clear of obstructions
3 Fire doors will be kept closed unless they are of the type which close automatically when the alarm sounds

Another example of a standard might be

Standard
Effective education for pain management is available some of the related criteria are

Criteria
1 Nursing staff have received instruction in pain management
2 There are written guidelines for symptom control available to nursing staff

A very different influence on standards in the United States has come from the introduction in some areas of a payment system based on Diagnosis Related Group (DRG) categories. These arose out of legislation passed under Public Law in 1983. To quote Franklin Shaffer (1988)

> the DRG is an attempt to define health care's various product lines. Each product line requires a specific set of outputs received by the patient. These outputs are defined in terms such as hours of nursing care, medications, laboratory tests, and diagnostic evaluations.

DRGs have then been used as a basis for determining the cost of care. The disease categories so determined are ascribed a cost which, in a system where the patient pays for the care he receives, will determine his treatment bill. However the system does allow those involved in care to become much more cost-conscious. The problem arises when it is assumed that cost-effectiveness and quality care are synonymous.

Where they have been introduced DRGs have had some considerable effect on nursing. Apart from making nurses much more cost-conscious it has had the effect of increasing early discharge of patients which in turn has increased the care which families have had to give in the home. Nurses have had much more than before to be involved in the education of families in order to help them cope with this situation.

As DRGs are based on a medical model the number of nursing hours calculated as required in any particular diagnostic category may well not be based on individual patient needs. Nurses have been required to be pro-active in this situation in order to maintain their position with regard to the patient.

One reaction to this by our American colleagues has been the introduction of Nursing Case Management. The nurse as case manager in this framework must ensure cost/quality outcomes for his/her patient. Nurses in this situation must not allow themselves to become victims of cost-containment but rather to use the situation to their advantage and make sure that a consideration of cost is part of their standard setting strategy.

We started at the beginning of this chapter to consider the factors which must be taken into account when thinking about 'structure' in standard setting. We have looked at the importance of manpower. There has also been a consideration of the resources within the environment of care and the way in which the support services within the organization work hand in hand with nursing in ensuring that the client has quality in the service offered at every level.

We did also suggest that it was not possible to consider structure standards in isolation and that they were inextricably linked with those of process and outcome. In the next chapter we will consider process standards and look at quality in action.

References

Ball J. A., Goldstone L. A., Collier M. M. (1984) *Criteria for Care – The Manual of the North West Staffing Levels Project.* Newcastle upon Tyne: Newcastle upon Tyne Polytechnic Products Ltd.

Canadian Nurses' Association (1966) Report on the project for the evaluation of the quality of nursing service. Canadian Nurses' Association, Ottawa. D.C.

Connor R. J. (1960) A hospital inpatient classification system. The John Hopkins University, Baltimore.

Department of Health and Social Security (1985) Performance Indicators Package DHSS, London.

Donabedian A. (1969) Some issues in evaluating the quality of nursing care. *American Journal of Public Health*, 59: **10** 1833–6.

East Dorset Health Authority (1987) Out-patient Standards, East Dorset Health Authority, Poole General Hospital, Poole.

English National Board (1989) Institutional and Course Approval/Re-approval Process, English National Board, London.

Gaither R. (1983) An Introduction to Quality Circles, The North Carolina Memorial Hospital, Chapel Hill, North Carolina.

George F. L., Kuehn R. P. (1955) *Patterns of patient care.* New York: Macmillan.

Giovannetti P. (1979) Understanding patient classification systems.

Journal of Nursing Administration, 9(2): 4–9.

Hyde P. (1984). *Implementing Quality Circles*, North Warwickshire Health Authority.

Joint Commission on Accreditation of Hospitals (1982) Accreditation manual for hospitals, Chicago: JCAH.

McKenzie R. (1979) Structural Standards Developing a service philosophy and a policy manual. *The Lamp*, 36 5–9.

National League of Nursing Education (1937) A study of nursing services in 50 selected hospitals. The United Hospital Fund of New York, New York.

North Warwickshire Health Authority (1984) Implementing Quality Circles, North Warwickshire Health Authority.

Nurses, Midwives, and Health Visitors Act (1979) HMSO.

Orlikoff J. E., Snow A. (1984) Assessing quality circles in health care settings: a guide for management, Chicago, Illinois: American Hospital Publishing Inc.

Salisbury Community Health Council (1987) Survey of Salisbury General Infirmary Outpatients, Salisbury Community Health Council, Old Manor Hospital, Salisbury.

Salisbury Health Authority (1988) Out-patient Standards, Salisbury Health Authority, Odstock Hospital, Odstock.

Shaffer F. A. (1988) DRGs: A new era for health care, Nursing Clinics of North America vol. 23, no. 3, September 1988.

Wessex Regional Health Authority (1989) Standards for nursing services in the Wessex region, Wessex Regional Health Authority, Highcroft, Winchester.

Will E. A. (1983) Quality Assurance in nursing. New Zealand Hospital, July, 1983 8–9.

Zander K. (1988) Nursing case management – resolving the DRG paradox. Nursing Clinics of North America vol. 23, no. 3, September, 1988.

5

The quality of care in action

In this chapter we will discuss setting standards and or criteria relevant to the process of nursing care, and some quality monitoring methodologies which predominately concentrate on process.

Process standards and criteria for nursing care as we indicated earlier are concerned with what nurses do and how they carry out care. They are a means of demonstrating the values, beliefs and knowledge of the profession and the individual nurse. The results of evaluating 'process' should enable the nurses to improve their practice in weak areas, discard that which is no longer relevant and reinforce that which is good.

As a profession we accept the notion of accountability. The United Kingdom Central Council (UKCC, 1984) in its pamphlet 'Code of Professional Conduct' emphasizes that the nurse is responsible and accountable for her/his actions. This isn't as easy to demonstrate as it would seem – given the debate about a definition of nursing, and the multifactorial input to care.

When we evaluate process standards we are looking at what the nurse does, but few instruments measure an individual nurse's responsibility for the quality that he/she personally gives. By the same token we cannot guarantee that the individual patient will benefit directly from an evaluation of the quality of the care he/she receives. We may have to accept that at this stage it is too difficult, logistically and ethically to implement such a system. It is our believe that if standards and criteria relevant to the patient could be put on the care plan, be correctly evaluated and have the facility to produce a quality score when necessary, this would go some way to over come the problem. Excelcare a system that uses care plans to individualize standards is discussed in Chapter 6.

Developing standards and criteria for the process of care

Definition

As we are concentrating on process perhaps we should look at a definition of nursing care – Phaneuf (1976a) says 'Nursing care is a process of interaction and transaction within which tasks and activities are carried out, but the care of the patient is more than the sum of the tasks and activities involved.' This seems to us a particularly useful definition for nurses when looking at process.

What does a nurse do?

It may also be useful to remind ourselves of some of the things a nurse does: comforts, advises, teaches, counsels, acts as an advocate, assesses patients needs, plans, implements and evaluates care, carries out procedures, prepares for and carries out the treatment prescribed by other professionals, adheres to rules and policies. Manages care, staff and resources. Maintains and enhances relationship with others, records and reports information. If nurses think about what they do and what they wish to achieve, it will guide them in selecting or devising a conceptual framework or needs list for developing process standards and criteria.

Care plans

If we accept that the nursing process is the framework that now guides nursing practice, then it is a good idea to look at care plans as a source of inspiration for process standards and or criteria. The nursing actions can indicate process standards. The goals of care can be a source of criteria for process, however to further confuse the issue these goals can also be a source of standards for outcomes.

Most process standards and/or criteria that are being produced focus on broad groups of patients and nurses, some nurses may decide to focus on one group of people with a particular condition or one aspect of care; for example: the condition diabetes and the treatment of varicose ulcers. The method of measuring may include: making observations of care in progress and the preparation of procedures, asking questions of staff, patients and people significant to him. It may also include checking records, and resources if they are relevant to what the nurse does.

Mason (1984) says 'Process standards define the quality of the implementation of nursing care.... A nursing intervention or procedure, contains the process standards that define actions done by the nurse to, for, or with the client'. Mason would seem to be advocating breaking nursing procedures down into standards to be used as the individual patient requires them. However it would be a mammoth undertaking to do this for all nursing procedures. Until all such procedures/standards can be put on a central computer to be selected for individual care plans, desirable though this method may be, it does not seem practical at present for all units. In the next chapter we discuss the Excelcare Nursing Care system which is Mason's method of setting and using standards which does use a computer to aid the work.

Research

We suggested in Chapter 3 that when developing standards it is useful to look for research on the subject that is to be evaluated, such work can indicate new concepts, areas of concern and or good practice all of which can give ideas for standard setting. Crow (1981) suggests that research 'may contribute to the choice of measures by (1) indicating what measure or measures may be used as a standard to judge or compare; and/or (2) by providing the background knowledge from which limitations or constraints in the use of that standard can be judged'. Some good sources of research material relevant to quality assurance are:

Nursing Research Abstracts, a quarterly journal produced by the Department of Health.

The Quality Assurance Abstracts produced by the King's Fund Centre and Published by the Library of the Department of Health.

The Nursing Quality Assurance Directory which is published jointly by the Royal College of Nursing and the King's Fund.

The Journal of Advanced Nursing and the International Journal of Nursing Studies.

Local and Regional Nurse Research Societies and Annual reports from Regional Health Authorities Research Committees.

The World Health Organization Regional Office for Europe also report their work on quality assurance. There are some quality assurance magazines being published and these together with the national and international nursing magazines can also be a source of research information and quality assurance. Nurses may also ask help and advice from their local librarian and investigate the possibility of carrying out a literature search on the relevant subject.

With this background in mind we offer some examples of standards and criteria

1 *Standard* (for recovery patient care). Position and movement carried out in safe and caring manner in accordance with the patient's physical state.

Critera: On repositioning the patient's head is properly supported.

On transferring patient's brakes are applied to the trolley/table and bed.

The above standard with criteria, of which there are 19, was devised by the National Association of Theatre Nurses (1987)

2 *Item* Nurse gives time to listen to conversation of patient or resident.

Cue: Eye to eye contact between nurse and patient is evident.
Sufficient time is allowed for patient to talk or respond.
The patient is allowed to finish sentence before the nurse leaves.

P. A. Nursing Quality Measurement Scale. (*this methodology does not use the word standard or criterion)

Standard: Each patient will have a written care plan which is relevant and up to date.

Criteria:
The care plan will be signed by the nurse when:
● prescribing care.
● reviewing care.
● discontinuing care.

The above standard was developed by the Nursing Standards Group, The General Unit, Salisbury Hospitals (1988). Salisbury Health Authority.

Because we are now going to be discussing some systems for evaluating nursing care and management; we feel we should say a little more about bias, a subject we touched on in Chapter 3. If we look at the word bias we see it means 'any special influence that sways the mind, a prejudice' (*Chambers Dictionary*, 1980). We obviously want the results from the evaluation procedure to be as accurate as possible. Therefore we have to acknowledge the factors that influence bias, so that we can try to do something about them. Some of these factors can be the choice of the wrong instrument to do the job or the inadequate preparation of people and the environment. They may include the Hawthorne effect which refers to the change in the subjects' behaviour because they know they are being observed, and the observer carrying out his/her task in an area in which he/she feel uncomfortable.

The relevant patients, staff and records may not be available. The way the questions are asked can influence results. Patients may not understand the questions or the reasons for them, and they may have forgotten the facts. Patients and nurses may give the answers they think the observer wishes to hear or on some occasions they may deliberately give incorrect answers.

The way the data is interpreted through lack of information, prejudice or knowledge. The person concerned may become tired and not complete the evaluation exercise correctly. The use of the 'non applicable' facility available in some instruments can be misinterpreted through inadequate knowledge or preconceived ideas.

What are the answers to these problems? We offer the following suggestions: Examine a number of quality monitoring methodologies before selecting one. Check that the standards and criteria are able to do what is required. Carry out a pilot study of the instruments. Have good communications, let staff know what is going on. Publicize quality assurance systems in patients' information sheets. Provide effective education and sufficient practice for staff. Use random selection of patients, ie everyone has a chance of being picked. Questions should be clearly phrased. Give back results of evaluation on time.

Have the quality monitoring methodology evaluated periodically perhaps every 18 months. Carry out inter–observer–

reliability testing at least once a year. Review the non applicable responses when the results are being correlated.

We must take whatever action we can to prevent bias occurring, although we cannot always guarantee that it will be successful. Bias can result in inaccurate high scores as well as inaccurate low scores, neither result being of use to anyone.

Selected quality monitoring methodologies:

Qualpac – the quality patient care scale by Wandelt and Ager (1974), is a development which began in 1966 at the College of Nursing, Wayne State University, USA, from the Slater Nursing Performance Rating Scale. Qualpac is a 68 item scale designed to measure nursing care received by patients in any setting, whilst the care is in progress. The 68 items are divided into six sections.

- psychosocial individual.
- psychosocial group.
- physical.
- general.
- communication.
- professional implications.

A Cue Sheet is provided to give specific examples to help define or clarify the 68 items. Patients are randomly selected. The number can be as few as five patients or 15% of the patients whichever is the greater. Ratings are carried out by the observers spending two hours in direct observation of the care being provided to the patient and approximately one hour auditing the nursing records.

The scoring is rated as best care through to poorest care along a five-point scale which yields a numerical score. 'The standard of measurement is care expected of a first level staff nurse' (Wandelt and Ager, 1974).

In examining the items and cues one cannot help being concerned at the number that call for value judgement, we also think some of the cues are ambiguous. It can be difficult choosing to which category of care the rating should be allocated. Does one always make the right judgement of best care, or between best and average care, or average care or between average and poorest care? It can also be difficult making a judgement if a lot of activities are occurring at the same time. A further area of concern is the length of time needed to observe care in one area.

Qualpac has been tested in a university and some hospitals in America. A report of the pretests and subsequent tests are recorded in the handbook which contains: the scale, instruction on how to use the scale including the education and inter–observer–reliability requirements, and the reasonings and philosophical concepts underlining the work; of particular interest is the section on judgement. The explanations go some way to answer the concerns we have highlighted.

Perhaps the most difficult area in which to set 'process' standards and to measure, are those aspects of care that demonstrates the nurses empathy and sensitivity for the patient. It is our opinion that Qualpac attempts to solve this difficulty. We feel that it is the best scale available for observing how nurses react to the needs of patients particularly in the area of communication, for example 'the infant is looked at and talked to as he receives a bottle feeding' (Wandelt and Ager, 1974).

We do have to remember that Qualpac was developed for American nurses, If British nurses wish to use it they must examine it to make sure it suits their culture and needs. Wiles and Wood (1985) reported on their experience in assessing Qualpac and the Nursing Audit, they conducted workshops for auditors and Qualpac assessors and Qualpac was assessed in clinical areas. It was concluded that 'The Qualpac scale ... appears to be a useful tool when undertaking concurrent evaluations of care. But some problems remain for instance, some items were never recorded by the assessors. There was also difficulty in establishing the exact meaning of some items and therefore, poor reliability in recording some observations.' However the participants of the workshops appeared to be positive about using quality monitoring scales. 'They were convinced that concurrent scales are useful in evaluating standards of care,' and interestingly, 'Not only were they able to pinpoint the strengths and weaknesses in the care given by other nurses, but they had an increased awareness of their own.' Qualpac does concentrate on patient care and although it can be fatiguing to use, it does produce a lot of facts about patient care and nurse behaviour.

We do not know of any published research on the use of the Qualpac in the UK.

The Phaneuf Nursing Audit was developed in America in the early 1960s by Phaneuf (1976b) 'It is a 50 item scale designed to measure retrospectively the quality of care received by a patient during a particular cycle of care'. The audit is carried out by an audit committee composed of nurses of varied experience who meet monthly to audit a number of randomly selected records of patients who have been discharged the previous month. The auditors look at the 50 items which are divided into seven nursing functions which serve as criteria:

1 the application and execution of doctor's legal orders
2 the observation of symptoms and reactions
3 supervision of the patients
4 supervision of those participating in care (except the doctor)
5 reporting and recording
6 the application of nursing procedures and techniques
7 the promotion of health by direction and teaching

Scoring is carried out by the rater making a choice of yes, no, uncertain or not applicable for every one of the 50 items, to which numerical values has been ascribed.

A disadvantage cited by van Maanen (1979) is 'that written reports are easily given too much weight and that judgement can be influenced by the quality of language skills rather than the real content of given nursing care'. We should bear this in mind if we develop our own instrument, perhaps we should not have too many standards or criteria that evaluate the documentation.

After each audit the committee submits a report with recommendations. The administrator responds in writing to the committee. It is said that such reports brings about change, without doubt if someone in a position of authority has to respond in this way to such a group, there is surely more chance of getting things done or receiving a credible explanation of why action is not possible.

Rush Medicus Quality Monitoring Methodology for Nursing Care is probably the best-known methodology to measure the quality of nursing care in the world. 'The project was originated in 1972 by the Medicus Systems Corporation of Chicago and the Rush Presbyterian–St Lukes Medical Center Chicago and the Baptist Medical Center in Birmingham, Alabama.' (Hegyvary and Haussmann 1975). The construct is based on nursing process, patient needs and provision of support services. The instrument is composed of six main objectives and 32 sub-objectives with a master criteria list of 357. Each sub-objective contains three to 26 criteria considered relevant to its evaluation. The criteria are available for medical, surgical, obstetrics emergency units, recovery rooms, psychiatry and the nursery which has an additional questionnaire for parents. A classication of patients according to their level of self-sufficiency is used. Each quality criterion in the methodology is coded to the type of patient to which it most likely applies.

Observation worksheets (questionnaires, i.e. part of the instrument) are generated from a computer with 30–50 observations to be evaluated. The specific configuration of criteria on any one worksheet is somewhat different from that of other worksheets for the same patient types – this reduces observer monotony and prevents staff from anticipating what is going to be evaluated. The sources of information are:

- patient record
- patient interview
- patient observation
- patient environment
- nurse interview
- nursing personnel observation
- observer inference
- unit (ward) management observation

Quality on any unit (ward) is monitored on a basis of 10 per cent of one month's patient admissions, three times a year. Observations are distributed randomly across days and times of day. 'The designers have produced a work book and an action plan to enable the necessary people to respond to the evaluation results. The designers also emphasize how important education and inter-observer-reliability training is in maintaining this methodology' (Kemp, 1983).

Haussmann and Hegyvary (1976) report that the instrument has had a great deal of statistical analysis, testing and refining, it was field tested in 19 hospitals in the USA. One of the conclusion is that 'extensive instrument testing and construct analysis demonstrate substantial reliability and validity for the quality monitoring system. van Maanen (1981) warns that whilst the methodology can make a significant contribution to the profession of nursing, it may be the most expensive in terms of resources.

Hegyvary (1979) writes 'it is suggested that the quality of the nursing process is subject to considerable variation as a result of influences from non-clinical system,' she also says 'although the nursing process is an appropriate focus for monitoring quality care, decisions about improving the quality of care must take into account the large scope of factors that may influence nursing practice.' However on examining the master criteria list there do not seem to be many support service criteria available, at least not as we in the UK understand the term. A weakness of the instrument is the scoring system, it is not easy to understand the reasoning behind the different numerical weights given to some responses.

We feel we can learn much from this methodology. 'The instrument appears easy to use' and 'the questions to aid the interpretation of the instrument are well constructed' (Kemp, 1983). The patient classification system which is part of this methodology is also used to aid manpower planning. We would like to be able to say that this methodology could be used in the UK, however we are not sure that the patient categorization system could transfer easily to this culture. The objectives are sound but some would need to be anglicized, the criteria would, with very few exceptions, need very few alterations. There would also need to be resources available to implement the methodology. However if we are routinely to monitor care perhaps we should invest in a system that is not fatiguing to observers, patients or significant others and has all the other benefits we have highlighted.

Monitor – an Index of the Quality of Nursing Care for Acute Medical and Surgical Wards which 'is an adaption for the United Kingdom of the Rush Medicus Nursing Process Methodology' (Goldstone, et al., 1984) Monitor consists of four separate patient-based questionnaires, each one relating to a different category of patient dependency, and a further ward-based questionnaire. Monitor is reported to 'have been researched in the UK on 26 acute medical and surgical wards within the North West Regional Health Authority' (Goldstone et al., 1984). The methodology involves the carrying out of pre-Monitoring preparation which includes setting up a steering group, involving care staff, consulting unions, professional organizations and the ethical committee, all of which is clearly explained in the Monitor manual. It is suggested that the instrument be used once a year. The entire population of a ward or twelve patients, three from each category randomly selected may be included in the evaluation procedure. Two assessors (observers) carry out the evaluation procedure. The number of observations to be made covers 60–140 according to the patients' dependency level. The source of information is gathered from nursing records, patient and nurse interviews, patient observation and observation of the environment. The observations are broadly grouped according to the stages of the nursing process.

The scoring system is well set out in the manual and easy to use, the responses have one of three possibilities; yes, no and not applicable. The final total gives an index of the quality of care for a ward, expressed in percentage form. The designers suggest 'a detached review by the assessors and the ward sister/charge nurse of the completed Monitor documents, of the specific scores, and especially those questions with multiple 'no' responses should, after appropriate discussion, lead to a strategy/training programme to correct those nursing inadequacies demonstrated in the no responses'.

It is of concern to us that there are so many questions/ observations to be made of and about one patient at any one time. Some observers may find patients are too ill to answer the number of questions being asked; for example there are 46 questions for category iii patient, those patients needing above average care, and 22 for category iv patient, those patients requiring maximum care. Nurses may find the document time consuming and tiring to use. It is a disappointment that Monitor questions are not in sub-sets as they are in the Rush Medicus Methodology.

Barnett and Wainwright (1987) in discussing Monitor highlight the difficulty of accepting the statement that the instrument can be used in task allocated wards as well as wards where staff use the nursing process. They point out that as the original instrument was meant to evaluate the nursing process and individualized care, 'any ward using task allocation would presumably receive a low rating. The tool cannot therefore be used with confidence in a task orientated setting, or to make comparisons between patient centred and task centred care, unless it is clearly understood that it is likely to be biased in favour of patient-centred care.'

Brittle and Marsh (1986) identify, as they see it, some of the limitations of Monitor including the concern over the use of the 'not applicable responses and the inadequate testing of inter-observer reliability'. Goldstone (1986) responds to these concerns by pointing out that there is a 'need to study the non applicable responses because they may deal with a substantial aspect of care on which no indicator has emerged. Additionally, it is always desirable, even with a score of 80% to check the remaining 20% as they could be vital and life threatening – or relatively unimportant' he then points out that Monitor 'indicates – it does not measure'. In referring to observer reliability Goldstone feels that 'if observers are prepared properly by discussing the meaning and their understanding of the questions in advance and familiarizing themselves with the documentation they will agree on a minimum of 90% questions for any patient. The average is agreement in over 95% of the questions'.

Whelan (1987) also expresses concern about bias, but feels that Monitor provides an easy and accessible method of measuring the quality of care. Hilton and Dawson (1988) identify the limitations and the positive aspects of using Monitor, one of the latter being, 'Monitor is a useful tool and has indicated achievements both in broad areas and in detailed aspects of care.'

There is now available Senior Monitor, Junior Monitor and Neuro Monitor, and District Nursing Monitor, a Monitor for health visiting and for midwifery is being developed. The developers of Monitor have also developed a patient categorization system which aids quality monitoring and nurse manpower planning, called 'Criteria for Care'. Table 5.1 is an example of a page taken from Monitor.

NATN Quality Assurance Tool has been developed in the UK from the mid 1980s onwards by The National Association of Theatre Nurses, the instrument is divided into five sections:
• preparation of personnel
• pre-operative patient care
• operating room care
• recovery patient care
• departmental organization.
The number of standards vary for each section and the number of criteria vary for each standard. On examining the tool one gets the feeling that this is a straightforward practical instrument

Table 5.1 REPRODUCED WITH THE PERMISSION OF NEWCASTLE UPON TYNE POLYTECHNIC PRODUCTS LTD.

	Patients											
	Code or Initials	6	7	8	9							

Patient's Emotional and Psychological well being is considered

Ask Patient

a DOES THE NURSE (OR OTHER STAFF, E.G. OCCUPATIONAL THERAPIST) DISCUSS WITH THE PATIENT HOW HIS ILLNESS MIGHT AFFECT HIS HOME SITUATION OR HIS WORK AND HELP TO PLAN HOW HE COULD COPE WHEN DISCHARGED?

To Patient: Has anyone talked to you about whether your illness might affect your home or work life and what to do about it?

No	
Yes	√
Not applicable/Not available	
57	
SCORE	1

Ask Patient

b DO THE NURSING STAFF INFORM THE PATIENT ABOUT ACTIVITIES BEFORE THEY ARE CARRIED OUT?

(Refers to routine care, not to written consent procedures)
To Patient: Do the nurses tell you what they are going to do before they give you some treatment, such as an injection or a dressing change?

No	
Yes	√
Not available/Not applicable	
58	
SCORE	1

Ask Nurse

c WHEN THE PATIENT'S CONDITION WARRANTS, DOES THE NURSE GIVE ATTENTION TO THE PATIENT'S NEEDS FOR DIVERSIONAL ACTIVITIES?

To Nurse: Do you think Mr/Ms _____ needs any diversional activities? If 'no' code 'Not applicable'. If 'yes', ask have any of the nursing staff arranged for diversional activities to be provided either by family or friends or by hospital staff?

No	
Yes sometimes	√
Yes usually	
Not applicable/Not available	
59	
SCORE	1

– the format is well set out and the scoring is stated simply. It is easy to see what is required of this tool. Many people designing their own instrument could benefit from using this style of presentation. However there is a danger that when an instrument is simple and easy to use that it may also be easy to manipulate the scores; because one can predict or remember what is going to be observed. This is something nurses have to keep in mind when using such instruments.

The designers recommend that an internal and external assessor should perform an annual review using the Quality Assurance Tool. They wisely say 'both assessors should have knowledge of theatre practice and be acceptable to operating theatre staff'. They also say that various parts of the tool can be used by a theatre sister or senior nurse to monitor aspect of care as they feel appropriate. It seems to us that a once-a-year evaluation is inadequate. It is a long time to wait to see if any changes made from previous monitoring have had any effect. There is also a danger that one can become complaisant or cynical knowing that an evaluation of the quality of practice will only take place annually.

The tool is reported to have been validated by a variety of hospitals around the country. The National Association of Theatre Nurses have a panel of people who will act as external assessors when needed. Apart from the advantages of having an outside assessor working with the local assessor, how comforting this must be for staff using the instrument for the first time, to have someone familiar with the methodology. The panel of assessors are also able to review and refine the tool when required and theatre nurses within the United Kingdom must surely benefit from this support system.

In reading the document which contains the tool. We were concerned that there is no mention of inter-observer reliability testing, or specific guidelines about education for the theatre staff. It is tempting to think that such education may not be necessary because the assessors are skilled in theatre practice and the clear framework of the tool. However if staff are going to have agreement on what they observe, and be in a position to analyse what is expected of them as well as their results, a well planned educational system is necessary. However the protocol recommends that before the annual review, the internal and external assessors discuss the Quality Assurance Tool and the procedure for carrying out the review with the operating depart-

Table 5.2 RECOVERY PATIENT CARE STANDARD 6 NURSE/PATIENT
COMMUNICATIONS ARE EFFECTIVE IN MINIMIZING FEAR, EMBARRASSMENT AND
ANXIETY.

SOURCE OF INFORMATION	CODE	CRITERIA	YES	NO	N/A
Observe	6.1	Verbal reassurance is directed to the unconscious patient	☐	☐	☐
Observe	6.2	There is tactile communication with the patient	☐	☐	☐
Observe Ask patient	6.3	When regaining consciousness the patient is reassured and orientated to his environment	☐	☐	☐
Observe Ask patient	6.4	The nurse informs the patient about activities before they are carried out	☐	☐	☐
Observe Ask patient	6.5	The nurse readily comforts an anxious or distressed patient	☐	☐	☐
Observe Ask patient	6.6	The nurse listens to the patient	☐	☐	☐
Observe Ask patient	6.7	The nurse responds promptly to the patients question and observations	☐	☐	☐
Observe Ask patient	6.8	The patients privacy is preserved within all practical limits	☐	☐	☐
Observe	6.9	The nurse anticipates the patients physical needs	☐	☐	☐
Observe	6.10	The nurse demonstrates a polite and caring attitude	☐	☐	☐
		SCORES:	☐	☐	☐
		NUMBER APPLICABLE:	☐		

DATE OF ASSESSMENT: _____

NAME OF INTERNAL ASSESSOR: _____

NAME OF EXTERNAL ASSESSOR: _____

$$\frac{\text{NUMBER SCORE YES}}{\text{NUMBER APPLICABLE}} = \text{_____} \times 100 = \text{_____ \% SCORE}$$

Reproduced with the permission of the National Association of Theatre Nurses mental staff. See Table 5.2 which is an example from one page of the tool: the fore-mentioned has ten criteria.

PA Nursing Quality Measurement Scale (1987). This scale has been developed by senior nursing consultants Flindall, Pearson, Binnie and a senior health care consultant M. McGreevy for P. A. which is a management consultancy organization. The designers have drawn ideas from a number of already established instruments. The purpose of this scale is to assess the overall quality of nursing care received by patients and residents in a variety of specialities. The tool is based on the premise that, irrespective of speciality, nursing has a core component. It is said to produce a descriptive judgement of quality and to give a numerical rating of quality. It is divided into five sections:

1 A profile of activity – ie workload and facilities.
2 Physical and human resources – this section is based on a standard of resources considered necessary by nurses to provide an effective nursing service.
3 The care process – this section focuses on the process of care both concurrently and retrospectively. It is in two parts, the first is an observation check list which is completed by observing total nursing care given to a group of four patients over a period of not less than two hours. Care is rated on a four-point scale leading to a final percentage score. The second part is a check list to apply to patients records. The assessors select 10 sets of records of recently discharged patients or of patients/residents who have received care for a minimum of three months in a long-stay setting
4 Is a questionnaire addressed to the patient/residents, significant others can answer for people who are unable to do this for themselves
5 Summary and recommendations in which the results of the whole scale are discussed and recommendations made. A grand total score is obtained. Two action plans are also provided which are a very important part of this methodology. The underlying premise of the scoring is that a 100% score denotes 'top quality' and less than 90% demands that care/resources be reviewed. It is very refreshing to find a methodology that will specify a desirable score and what percentage requires corrective action.

The work book is well presented, the instructions on how to carry out the calculation for the scoring is easy to understand and appears easy to use. However there is no mention of the action needed for the 'not applicable' responses.

The nursing management consultants provide comprehensive in-service training and put emphasis on preparation of staff which includes quality assessment, analysis and presentation of findings to both nursing and general management. We do have some unease about the lack of comment on inter-observer (assessors) reliability training and testing – although 'the third day of the three day course is spent in the wards to allow the assessors to practise under supervision' (PA, 1988). The observations in this scale cover a good cross section of care but some of the observations to be made from the record seem to us to be ambiguous. A further concern is the number of questions to ask the patient/resident or their advocate, there are 42 in number and one wonders whether this is too many for some patients.

The check sheet for the patient care observation is well presented and cues give concise guidance for most of the items, leaving little to subjective judgement. This methodology is being used in some units in the UK but as yet has not been evaluated by research methods but we are told this is being planned for the future.

Wylie (1989) reports on the use of the PA Scale in the Ulster Hospital and says 'according to those responsible, the PA Scale has proven straightforward to administer, and it has the virtue of providing data speedily from assessors who have the respect of their peers.' However she does also point out that 'the scale requires a lot of direct observation of care. The assessors observe care given to a group of patients, during a period of not less than two hours.' She concludes 'overall the information from the survey stood up well as a foundation for working out improvements for quality of care.'

We have been unable to show examples of some of the instruments we have discussed for copyright reasons or we have been unable to obtain permission to reproduce the work. However all the works we have mentioned have been described by their authors and most are available in large nursing libraries. It should also be remembered that most workbooks that accompany the different methodologies contain research data relevant to that methodology.

There are performance appraisal systems used in the Health Service that monitor staff performance including peer review. The standards used may have been devised by the professional organizations, educational bodies, employees and or employers. We decided not to discuss such systems, choosing instead to focus on patient care – however it can be argued that perform-ance standards should be part of any chapter on the process of nursing. We hope our readers will forgive us for having just 'homed in' on patient care standards. In the next chapter we will be discussing the results of care on the patient or those significant to him.

References

Barnett D., Wainwright P. (1987) Between two tools. *Senior Nurse*. vol 6. no 4. April. 40–2.

Brittle, J., Marsh J. (1986) Definition or measurement? *Nursing Times*. November 5. 36–7.

Chambers Twentieth Century Dictionary (1980) Ed. Macdonald A. M. Edinburgh: W. R. Chambers Ltd.

Crow R. A. (1981) Research and the standards of Nursing Care: What is the relationship? *Journal of Advanced Nursing*, **6** 491–6.

Goldstone L. (1986) A pointer to quality. *Nursing Times*. November 5 38–9.

Goldstone L. A., Ball J. A., Collier M. M. (1984) Monitor – An index of the quality of nursing care for acute Medical and Surgical wards. Newcastle upon Tyne, England: Newcastle upon Tyne Polytechnic Products Ltd.

Haussmann R. K. D., Hegyvary S. T. (1976) Field testing the nursing quality monitoring methodology Phase 11. *Nursing Research*. September–October. vol 25. no. 5. 324–31.

Hegyvary S. T., Haussmann R. K. D. (1975) Monitoring Nursing Care Quality. *Journal of Nursing Administration*, June 17–26.

Hegyvary S. T. (1979) Nursing Process: the basis for evaluating the quality of nursing care. *International Nursing Review*, 26, **4**. 113–6.

Hilton I., Dawson J. (1988) Monitor evaluated. *Senior Nurse*, **8(5)**, 10–11.

Kemp N. Quality Assurance Programmes and the Nursing Process. Smith and Nephew/Florence Nightingale Scholarship, 1983. Florence Nightingale Committee, London.

Mason, E. W. (1984) *How to write Meaningful Nursing Standards*. 2nd edn. New York: John Wiley and Sons Ltd.

P. A. (1987) Nursing Quality Measurement Scale. PA Consulting

Services, Ltd. Knightsbridge. London.
Phaneuf M. A. (1976a) Quality assurance: a nursing view. *The New Zealand Nursing Journal.* February, p. 10.
Phaneuf M. (1976b) *The Nursing Audit – Self Regulation in Nursing Practice,* 2nd edn. (1976) New York: Appleton–Century–Croft.
UKCC United Kingdom Central Council for Nursing Midwifery and Health Visiting. (1984) Code of Professional Conduct for the Nurse Midwife and Health Visitor. UKCC London.
Rush Medicus – Nursing process quality monitoring instrument. (1974) Public Health Service Control No 1, Nu-24299. United States Department of Health, Education and Welfare. Washington D.C. 20402.
van Maanen. H. M. Th. (1979) Perspectives and problems on quality of nursing care: an overview of contributions from North America and recent developments in Europe. *Journal of Advanced Nursing.* **4.** 377–89.
van Maanen H. M. Th. (1981). Improvements of quality of nursing care: a goal to challenge in the eighties. *Journal of Advanced Nursing* **6.** 3–9.
Wandelt M. A. and Ager J. W. *Quality Patient Care Scale* (1974) New York: Appleton–Century–Crofts.
Wainwright P., Burnip S. (1983) Qualpacs at Burford. *Nursing Times.* February 2. 36–8.
Wiles A., Wood K. (1985) More about Qualpacs. *Nursing Times.* Jan 2. 51–2.
Wylie M. (1989), Quality Assurance, Bulletin No 14. Ulster Hospital Unit of Management. 31st March.

Useful Addresses

Debra Unsworth
Department of Health, Nursing Research Librarian
Room 94, Hannibal House
Elephant and Castle
London, SE1 6TE

National Association of Theatre Nurses
22, Maint Parade
Harrogate
North Yorkshire
HG1 1BV

6

Evaluating the results of care

In this chapter we focus on the setting of standards and criteria that relate to outcome. We also report on the debate that concerns the relationship between outcome and other areas of evaluation, and will discuss some methodologies that use outcome standards to measure patient care.

Outcome evaluation as Donabedian (1969) says 'consists of the assessment of the end results of care usually specified in terms of patient health, welfare and satisfaction.' Outcome can be seen as the most worthwhile of all the measures, because it should indicate if care has been successful or not. It is also the most difficult area in which to set nursing care standards, for many reasons. It is not easy to identify outcomes which are the results of nursing intervention alone. Patient care is usually multidisciplinary, therefore who can say who influenced the outcome, it may also be influenced by the patient's own ability to meet the requirements of health care. The patient's expectation may be different from the standard being measured, and/or his level of understanding may not enable him to make a judgement about care. Nursing responsibility is not always 'clear cut', and people significant to the patients may have a greater effect on his health state than any professional can hope for.

It is essential to quantify the outcomes of care, to ensure that patients, the community, the profession and the individual nurse are satisfied with what is accomplished. There is a need to ensure that nurses are seeing patients as individuals whose uniqueness is given attention, whatever their reason for receiving care. It is also necessary to check that we are not wasting valuable resources and using ineffective procedures.

Some outcomes of health statistics have been measured for many years, for example levels of mortality, morbidity, and disability. Measuring the results of care may highlight areas that need further attention and the need for change, it can also provide the chance to acknowledge good things and to give some praise. The results of outcome measurement can further nursing knowledge and should maintain or enhance public confidence in the profession.

Setting outcome standards and criteria

Outcome standards for our purpose centre on the patient. They may involve changes in or maintenance of his physical, mental and spiritual health, his social wellbeing, and can include knowledge, learning behaviour, motivation, self care skills and satisfaction with what is being accomplished.

We discussed in Chapter 3 the preparation for standard setting and criteria development and the characteristics of standards and criteria which of course also apply to outcomes. In Chapter 5 to help us set process standards, we asked the question, what nurses do? In this chapter we should ask the question – what are the desired results of what nurses do? and what does the patient want from his care?

The patient care plan, as we have said previously, is a good source of standards and criteria. The goal statements will be of particular help in indicating what the standard might be.

Standards can be written as outcome standards with outcome criteria, for example:

Standard: All patients are at all times treated courteously.

Criteria: The patient was treated courteously on admission to the ward? Ask patient, 'When you were admitted to the ward were you treated courteously?'

> The patient is included in the conversation that takes place in his/her presence
> Ask patients, 'Are you included in the conversation, when nurses give you care?'
> The patient is called by his/her preferred name?
> Check care plan and ask patient 'do all the nurses call you by the name you prefer?'
> (if the answer is sometime or some do/some do not – code no)

Standards can also be written as a general standard statement with an outcome criterion or criteria, for example.

Standard

Clients attending the day centre are given the choice of participating in social activities.

Criterion

The individual feels he/she can decline to take part in any activity if he/she wishes.

Ask client 'do you feel you can refuse to take part in any activity that's going on?'

A framework or nursing model will guide the standard setting, but remember a lot of helpful suggestions can be obtained from the patients and patient interest groups, surveys and research studies. If you are stuck and not able to think what to write it is also helpful to think of your own experience of care, or that of someone close to you; this may seem unscientific, but it often reminds one of things that are important to patients.

An outcome standard may be difficult to set because of the time factor; it may not be easy to evaluate because of the problem of predicting when it will be achieved. A criterion may take some time to become apparent, indeed it may not become apparent until after the patient has left the health care setting.

Developing criteria for outcomes

Outcome criteria will enable the standard to be measured. The kind of things that the criteria could indicate are: Is the patient's physical status improving? Is the patient comfortable? Is he free of pain? Do the nurses treat the patient correctly? Are staff courteous and kind without being patronizing? Did they show empathy and sensitivity for his condition? Are procedures carried out effectively (from the patient's point of view)? Is the patient given sufficient information? Is the patient comfortable in the environment? Does the patient, if he chooses to, feel that he is involved in decision making about his care? Are communications good? Are the patient's family and/or friends treated courteously? Are cultural and social needs acknowledged and met to the patient's satisfaction? Is the patient able to practise his religion without difficulty or embarrassment? Above all is the patient made to feel valued?

How to measure outcomes

If we say outcomes are the results of nursing care, then it is evident that to measure them one needs to ask the patient what he thinks about his care. As we have pointed out he may not have the understanding or knowledge about certain procedures or treatments or even wish to think about the subject. There are also times when observation will be the most appropriate method of carrying out evaluation, for example, the decreasing size of a pressure sore or a change in behaviour. Outcome information may also be obtained from reports or the patient care record.

The methods for measuring quality of nursing care outcomes may include:

Lists of standards and criteria are the most usual method of evaluating quality, for example most of the instruments referred to in the previous chapter use the list approach. The disadvantage of criteria listing is that the criteria will be used for all patients in the selected population whether it is appropriate or not.

Interview is a useful method for obtaining information not easily acquired by observation. This may be conducted with the patient or on occasions the patient's advocate. There may be times when people other than the advocate who are significant to the patient will be asked questions, when for instance he is not able to answer for himself; however there is an ethical problem here – does it suit the patient that we ask others who are not professional carers about his care?

If members of other disciplines are to be interviewed, they should be cognisant of the quality assurance programme. Training is required if interview techniques are to be successful.

Observation of care may include observing the patient's physical status and behaviour. One of the disadvantages is observer bias which we discussed in the previous chapter.

Questionnaires completed by the patient can indicate outcomes, but where and when this is done may have an effect on the results. Some patients may not be inclined to answer questions about their health care experience whilst they are still a patient in hospital. This does seem to us to suggest that retrospective evaluation of care after discharge could produce some worthwhile information, unfortunately such techniques can be costly to implement.

Surveys are a type of non-experimental research which can be carried out by observation, interview or questionnaire or a combination of all three. They give an indication of the patients' satisfaction with the facilities and care being offered. An area where surveys are often used is in out-patient departments.

Audit groups may measure outcomes of care by checking the records either concurrently or retrospectively against a list of standards and or criteria. How innovatory it would be if patients were invited to attend such groups to discuss their care!

Scales of outcome criteria, in which the patient grades the criteria in order of importance or selects a rating according to his own experience. These activities can be carried out using a list or points on a continuum.

Criteria maps, which are different in formation and conceptual approach from criteria lists, will be discussed on page 88.

Example of standards
Standard
(based on the need, safe environment)
The patient does not come to any harm whilst in hospital.

Data Source	Criteria:
Nursing record & handover	The risk of developing pressure sores is assessed for each individual patient
Observation	the relief of pressure is achieved by appropriate nursing action, eg lifting, turning, positioning, early mobilization and the use of special equipment, eg, beds, mattresses, pillows.

Nursing record & handover	The integrity of the patient's skin is evaluated at least once daily.
Observe patient	*Outcome* The patient does not develop a pressure sore.

The fore-mentioned standard was developed by nurses of the Orthopaedic unit, Queen Alexandra Hospital, Portsmouth (1989). The standards focus on patient outcomes. The standard setting group send out samples of the standards and criteria they have developed to all the orthopaedic wards in the unit for comments and as the beginning of a validation process. This work is in the very early stages.

Standard (based on the Need-Control by the patient)
Residents influence decision making.

Criteria
Residents are involved in discussions about their care. Residents feel able to have a say in the organization of ward activities which affects them (Nattrass, 1989). Quality of life for elderly people in longer term care. (Unpublished work. Wessex Regional Health Authority)

Standards

(Problem – difficult breathing).

Standard statement: The patient who has difficulty breathing is supported and monitored for deterioration or complications of his or her problem.

Outcome standards:

1 Within four hours activities that increase difficulty were identified.
2 The patient states he/she received assistance with the activities that increased difficulty breathing.
3 The doctor was notified immediately if:–
   - amount and character of sputum altered
   - increased breathlessness

chest pain
tachycardia
hypertension
restlessness
anxiety
hypoxia
hypercapnia
confusion
stupor

4 Patient states that at all times he/she was in a comfortable position which helped him/her breath more easily'.

The previous standard was developed by the nurses of West Dorset Health Authority (1988) – they use process, outcome and content standard as part of their quality monitoring methodology. This standard statement also has six process standards (Unpubished work, Standards of Care Project. West Dorset Health Authority).

The process/outcome debate

We have some reservations about whether it is possible to validate nursing practice by just looking at outcome – is there not a danger that the outcome will be positive but the practice may not be as the patient or the profession would wish? A person may make a good recovery from a stroke – learn to walk again, and can with some help feed himself, he also dresses without help but the patient may not be asked, or it may not be observed if the nurses always changed his jacket if he spilled his food, if he was left sitting on the commode too long or whether he was given a mouth wash because his mouth was dry. The patient does not usually know what care was missed or the phone messages he did not receive or if his diet was adequate for his needs! We also of course have to keep in mind that other factors will have influenced this person's recovery.

Luker (1981) cites Bloch's observation about process and outcome evaluation: 'In process evaluation one examines and makes judgement about what is done by the care provider. In outcome evaluation one examines and makes judgement about the achievement of patient-orientated objectives. The result of the latter however, can be dangerously sterile, because when process is not also examined one cannot know what caused the favourable or unfavourable outcomes. Only evaluation which encompasses both process and outcome has the potential for great impact on the quality and care.' It is further suggested that 'the interventions which most frequently produced a favourable outcome might be identified and subsequently used to replace those interventions which most frequently produced an un-favourable outcome.' This should of course be one of the advantages of monitoring nursing care quality.

Hegyvary and Haussmann (1976) conducted a study which looked at aspects of the nursing process and patient care outcomes in three dimensions predicted to be related to nursing care: physical condition, psychological status and health knowledge. The researchers chose patients suffering from congestive heart failure and patients undergoing abdominal hysterectomy. The conclusions were 'these findings suggest that the relationship between the nursing process and patient outcomes is somewhat inconsistent and may differ with various types of patients. The focus on outcome assessment is supported, as in every type of outcome with both types of patients, some part of the nursing process showed a significant correlation'. They concluded 'the data suggests that limiting quality assessment to either process or outcome measures may be inappropriate because of the inconsistency of the relationship and the lack of conclusive evidence regarding causes and effects'. This seems to be what many researchers are saying and what many of us instinctively feel.

McAuliffe (1978 & 1979) has reviewed some studies on process and outcome evaluation in medical care. It seems to us they are facing the same problems as nursing. Writing in 1978, he says 'since the validity of outcome measures has never been determined, there is little reason at present for believing that outcome measures are more valid than process measures'. In 1990 the position doesn't seem to have changed. We should perhaps think about the following statement, 'No regulatory body can insist that patient outcomes be positive, nor do positive outcomes insure that care was appropriate or skilful' (McAuliffe, 1979). The reader who is concerned about this subject will find Openshaw's (1984) Literature Review interesting and helpful.

Donabedian (1969) in discussing the differing opinions about whether to use structure, process or outcome to evaluate, points out that which is used depends 'on the nature of the agencies' responsibility and questions the agency feels required to ask', he further points out that 'a well rounded system of quality appraisal would probably include concurrent or coordinated assessment of structure, process and the end results, to the extent that each of these is observable and measurable under the constraints inherent in any given setting'.

Quality monitoring methodologies for measuring patient care outcomes

Few established quality measuring methodologies have focused entirely on the outcome of care for many reasons some of which we have identified previously. However some of the professional nursing organizations around the globe have attempted to set outcome standards and or criteria. The American Nurses Association (ANA) have been involved in quality assurance since the mid 1960s and have published standards for various nursing specialities. Jacquerye (1984) writes that 'to comply with the Federal requirement for Professional Standards Review Organization (PSRO) the ANA specially recommend use of outcome criteria and the retrospective approach.'

Kitson (1989) writing about professional nursing organizations and standard setting points out 'the majority of work has gone into the development of process standards based on the nursing process methodology, but organizations such as the RANF (Royal Australian Nursing Federation) have been successful in systematically identifying a range of structure process and outcome standards for nursing'. Our own Royal College of Nursing as we mentioned earlier have developed the dynamic standards setting approach which suggests using a standard statement and criteria based on structure process and outcomes. It will be interesting to see what research studies make of these methods.

Criteria maps developed by Greenfield et al. (1978) are based on branching logic. They are being used by some doctors in the UK, 'The method consists of sets of explicit criteria for a specific condition usually beginning with a presenting sign and symptom. Depending on the presence/absence or degree of any symptom, it determines which branch shall be followed in an attempt to follow the decision steps of the physician' (cited by Openshaw, 1984). We have mentioned criteria maps because it seems a logical way of examining outcomes of care. It would also seem to be a method that could benefit undividual patients, and perhaps demonstrate the decision making skills of individual practitioners. Table 6.1 is an example of a criteria map reproduced with the permission of Geraldine Padilla.

We have no experience of the following two projects, however we have decided to write about them, because we feel they could be of interest and value to nurses.

Padilla and Grant (1982) reported on their project to develop a methodology for evaluating the quality of nursing care as part of a quality assurance programme for nursing. The focus of the project is on patients who are suffering from cancer. An interesting aspect of this work and a marked change for nursing is the use of a conceptual framework, in this case Orem's theory of self care, together with the criteria map approach. Orem's model 'emphasizes the importance of decisions in the selection of process criteria, based on patient status and problems – the outcome criteria using this model is self care. . . . The mapping approach identifies problems which must be assessed and for which nursing must prescribe the actions and specifics relevant to patient outcome goals, . . . and permits evaluation of the correctness of nursing decisions given specific patient states or problems and the relationship between the selected interventions and actual patient outcomes.' Padilla and Grant (1982).

This project is obviously a big undertaking; it involves developing standards and criteria across agencies who care for people with cancer and protocols to implement and maintain the system. Perhaps the results from this work will reinforce the advantages of using a model of nursing for standards of care. Criteria maps appear to encourage logical thought, and emphasizes the importance of making the right decisions. This approach may also resolve the debate about the difficulty of evaluating process separate from outcome and vice versa. It will be interesting to follow the progress of criteria maps. This evolutionary approach heralds exciting times and a lot of hard work.

Patient Indicators of Nursing Care, sometimes referred to as PINK, and devised by Majesky et al. (1978) is a 24-item tool designed to measure quality of nursing care, which according to the authors, 'means the prevention of nursing care complications. Nursing accountable complications are seen as the presence of negative patient care outcomes as evidenced by observable physiological indicators. A negative outcome results when either the observed indicator which was present on admission remains evident up to seven days post admission or an absent indicator

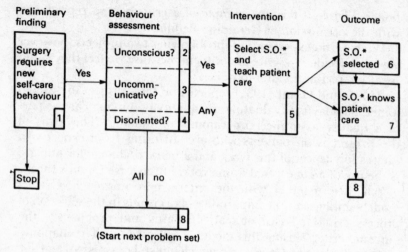

Table 6.1 SPECIFIC EXAMPLE OF A CRITERIA MAP PROBLEM SET

Reference for this example of a criteria map: Padilla, G. V. Quality Assurance Program for Cancer Nursing. In Evaluation Model for Innovative Care Programs Symposium. Western Society for Research in Nursing Conference, 1984 (Table 3).

becomes evident during this time period'. The indicators cover infection, immobility, and fluid imbalance which were broken down into items.

The tool is based on D. Johnson's conceptual framework which the researchers see as an appropriate model for their purpose. The list of 24 items is said to take approximately 15 minutes to administer and is easy to use. It takes place within the first 48 hours of the patient's admission, and then between five and seven days post admission. Scoring takes into account the conditions which have not changed as well as those that have. The work has had repeated pilot testing and was tested in four health care settings and an independent test was carried out to establish inter-rater reliability. 'The tool was found to be valid and reliable and to discriminate between long-term patients and patients with acute short-term elective surgery' (Majesky et al., 1978). The authors see the prevention of complications as a major responsibility of nursing. The focus of this study is on physical indicators, the authors admit that this limits their study. The tool does seem useful for monitoring a patient's physical status however it is worrying to think nurses are holding themselves accountable for some of these complications. We pose the question, would evaluating quality be easier if it was a multidisciplinary effort?

Excelcare Nursing System (Price Waterhouse, 1987) 'Is a micro computer based decision support system for planning, documenting, staffing, evaluating and costing nursing services based on nursing standards', and is said to be applicable to hospital and community care. The system is co-owned by Judith Daugherty and Elizabeth Mason two nurses working in the United States of America. The methodology for setting standards is based on Mason's 1984 work, which is clearly explained in her book *How to Write Meaningful Nursing Standards*.

Price Waterhouse is the organization who acts as agents in the United Kingdom for Excelcare. The nursing standards are developed in the domain of process, content and outcome using the framework of the nursing process. 'Standards are determined at the local level and validated in terms of producing positive outcomes before implementation. . . . The nursing standards on which the system is based are clustered into "Units of Care", related to the needs, problems or nursing diagnosis of the patient.' (Price Waterhouse, 1987).

Before we focus on the standard setting we would like to say something about the sections concerned with 'costing of the nursing service' and 'the staffing and assignment tool', because we feel it is relevant to quality and it is an important and useful part of this system.

The costing of the nursing service. For each patient entered into the system costs are developed according to the care planned and delivered. Each intervention listed under the Units of Care is assigned a time value, which enable costs to be made for direct and indirect nursing time. The hospital may choose to retain the values that have already been validated by Excelcare and are included in the system, or revalidate their own time standards. The authors do point out that indirect care can vary dramatically between hospitals and they do encourage an individualized evaluation of indirect care standards.

The staffing and assignment tool. 'Excelcare stores, compiles and updates the care plan data information after computing direct and indirect nursing time and costs' (Price Waterhouse, 1987). It is our opinion that the Excelcare nursing system, with its focus on units of care, and the care plan has the potential to sort out the ever present problem of skill mix.

Using the system for patient care. Mason (1984) defines a unit of care as 'the cluster of process, outcome, and content standards that define the nursing care for a given nurse diagnosis, health problem, or need; a desirable point on the health–illness continuum; or a specific developmental stage'.

Planning: After the assessment, the patient's problems/needs are identified as units of care. The nurse then accesses Excelcare, establishes a patient file and puts in the units of care. The nurse prints the care plan which she further individualizes for the patient. This entire process is said to take one minute when staff are familiar with the system.

Intervention/observation: The nurse uses the patient's care plan to give care. If a care plan is reproduced each day and stored in the Medical Record which it must be, because it is part of the primary medical record, and as such is available for future health care and legal purposes, an obvious consideration here is the amount of paper that may be generated and stored. It also may cost more than our present care plan material. Nurses must also be aware that if information is reproduced without much effort then it may not be read – we hasten to add that we do not think that expending a lot of effort necessarily produces good results!

Evaluation: At the end of each shift the nurse evaluates the care provided for the patient, afterwards at the microcomputer the nurse makes any revision to the care plan; finally a new plan is printed for each patient so a report can be given to the nursing staff on the next shift. There must be concern about the plan being changed on the computer. The information that has been changed should be saved so that the care plan is an accurate the true record of care that has been planned and given. It is essential that nurses using the microcomputer are aware of the danger of losing or erasing information that may be needed for care and legal purposes. Health districts wishing to use this system obviously need to make an investment of money to buy the computers and the software, and time and educational resources to give the necessary instruction and practice.

We are impressed with the way this system uses the framework of the nursing process, we feel it solves the problem of how patients benefit as individuals from quality monitoring. Nurses, are able to choose standards that have been devised and or validated for their areas. This method should save nursing time and should increase knowledge, and it is a continuous process of monitoring quality which has to be good for us all.

The standards

Previously we have talked about structure, process and outcome and commented upon Mason's approach to setting process standards. In her work she also uses 'Content' standards which she defines as 'the substance of nursing care that is communicated to others and the substance of the nurses' decisions.' Content standards cover such things as teaching patients and significant others, communications, multidisciplinary conferences/ meetings, data that must be recorded about the client and nursing care of the client and data that must be reported to other members of the nursing and health teams.

Outcome standards as defined by Mason (1984) is 'the expected change in the health status and environment following nursing care and the extent of the client's satisfaction with the nursing care. Both positive and negative outcomes result from nursing care. Positive outcomes occur when the care is appropriate to the client's needs. Good nursing care can also prevent negative outcomes for the client. Thus outcome standards describe the absence of negative outcomes as well as the presence of positive outcomes.' Mason also feels 'outcome standards should be developed for all nursing interventions and units of nursing care'. She suggests that there are three components of an outcome standard: the expected outcome, when the outcome occurs and how the outcome can be detected. This is a concise and very useful guideline to keep in mind when attempting to set outcomes.

A large number of generic units of care are available in the Excelcare system and may be validated for local use. Standards are also developed and validated by local staff 'To guarantee quality, every standard must be valid – that is, nursing care administered according to the standard must result in positive outcomes for clients. A standard is not valid unless it includes the criteria to evaluate the quality of nursing care. . . . Valid standards are precise, their meaning is shared by those who implement them and those who write them' (Mason 1984).

Example of an outcome standard

The absence of avoidable injuries to the clients legs and feet as indicated by an absence of the following:

1. Wounds or a break in the continuity of the skin
2. Burns
3. Callouses or corns
4. Ecchymosis

In Mason's (1984) book, the suggestions for writing standards are set out in steps, which are easy to understand and the results are free of ambiguity. The standards and criteria are not separate, which for some standards could be difficult to compose particularly, if requiring a yes or no response to quantify a quality score. The book contains exercises to enable nurses to test their understanding of this method of standard setting.

The Quality Monitoring Tool. 'Each unit of care is designed to include outcome standards. Periodically upon command, the computer generates check lists which can be used to measure compliance to each outcome standard. . . . This application allows the nurse manager to track quality levels with respect to staffing.' It is claimed that the manager can effectively reduce or increase staffing while monitoring the impact and that the system can therefore become part of an overall quality assurance programme, Price Waterhouse (1987). The approach used in this system sounds ideal, however, we are required to produce evidence, be it a numerical score, about what level of quality is being achieved and although this may be a narrow view the reality is that we are in a competitive culture where numbers count. We cannot find how quality scores are produced or demonstrated. However a great deal of work has gone into this system to try to solve many of the difficulties that are facing nurses today.

Excelcare nursing system covers many aspects of nursing care and management and we have only reported briefly on the system. Price Waterhouse do offer the services of nursing consultants to help with the implementation and training in the system and they provide fully documented user and orientation manuals.

We have discussed setting standards for structure process and outcome separately, however we feel that all three should be combined in one methodology. We have also appraised a number of quality monitoring methodologies, but the reader must be left to make up his own mind whether to choose one of those or to create his own. Whilst we have in this book focused on quality assurance for nursing let us not lose sight of the fact that all disciplines are working to the same ends – that of effective and good care, and let us hope that soon we will be able to pool our expertise for the benefit of all.

References

Donabedian A. (1969) Some Issues in Evaluating the Quality of Nursing Care. *American Journal of Public Health*. vol 59, no 10. October. 1833–6.

Greenfield S., Kaplan S. H., Goldberg G., Nadler M., Deigh-Hewertson R. (1978) Physician preference for criterion mapping in medical care evaluation. *Journal of Family Practice* **6**. 1079–86.

Hegyvary S. T., Haussmann R. K. D. (1976). The Relationship of Nursing Process and Patient Outcomes. *Journal of Nursing Administration*, November, 18–21.

Jacquerye A. (1984) Choosing a method of quality assurance. In *Measuring the Quality of Care. Recent Advances in Nursing.* (Willis L. D., Lindwood M. E. *ed*). Edinburgh: Churchill Livingstone, pp. 107–19.

Kitson A. L. (1989) The role of the professional organization in setting standards for nursing. Vard. 1 *Norden* vol 14. Arg. 9., 13–23.

Kitson A. (1986) The methods of measuring quality. *Nursing Times*. August 27. 32–34.

Luker K. A. (1981) An overview of evaluation research in nursing. *Journal of Advanced Nursing*. **6**. 87–93.

Majesky S. J., Brester M. H., Nishio K. T. (1978). Development of a Research Tool: Patient Indicators of Nursing Care. *Nursing Research*. November–December. vol 27, no 6. 365–71.

McAuliffe W. E. (1978) Studies of Process–outcome Correlations in medical care evaluations: a critique. *Medical Care*. November, vol xvi, no 11. 907–30.

McAuliffe W. E. (1979) Measuring the Quality of Medical Care: Process versus Outcome. Milbank Memorial Fund Quarterly/*Health and Society*. vol 57. no 1. 118–52.

Mason E. W. (1984) *How to write Meaningful Nursing Standards*. 2nd edn. New York: John Wiley & Sons Ltd.

Openshaw S. (1984) Literature Review: measurement of adequate care. *International Journal of Nursing Studies*. vol 21. no 4. 295–304.

Padilla G. V., Grant M. M. (1982) Quality assurance programme for nursing. *Journal of Advanced Nursing*. **7**. 135–45.

Price Waterhouse (1987) Excelcare – Nursing Management Information System. Bristol, England.

7

Educating for quality

In this final chapter we would like to explore the need for education, the selection of educational approaches which have been used in introducing quality assurance in various settings, and give some practical guidance to those who are involved in preparing staff to take part in a quality assurance programme. The credibility of such a programme does rest to a large extent on the preparedness of staff who participate in it.

There is concern amongst nurses that new ideas are introduced without staff being adequately prepared or even informed of the implications for them. There are times too, when the expectations of managers are unrealistic given the innumerable pressures put on clinical staff in these days of high bed occupancy and rapid throughput of clients. If you are reading this book then you are concerned about standards and quality; it should go without saying that you would want the scheme which you are involved with, at whatever level, to be produced and used with the greatest expertise possible.

The introduction of quality assurance into a health district is no mean task. It is something which in time will affect the working of everyone in the district. Success does not come easily, but then anything which is worthwhile very rarely does. In seeking to enable nurses to look critically at the standard of care which they are giving to their patients we may be asking them to come to terms with new terminology, and use new procedures with which they are unfamiliar.

Once standards are set then there may be a need to change practices which were once familiar and comfortable to improve the quality of care being provided. Change is never easy and the more radical it is the more difficult it is for people to make it fit with their presently held beliefs. The more uncertainty there is about change, the more people feel anxious and the lower their morale. If change is to be effective and long-lasting then we have to ensure that we have provided adequate support in the way of education and training, although this is only one kind of support which is needed.

Managers who are involved in the implementation of quality assurance schemes must be sure that their educational colleagues are involved so that from the beginning the process of change is facilitated by the provision of adequate and appropriate information and educational input. It does mean that educationists must themselves keep abreast with change in the clinical setting so that together they can take the scheme forward.

To quote the Oxford Health Authority's training brochure on Training for Quality:

'Experience from many successful companies in the private sector shows that if quality initiatives are to be effective in the long run, staff at all levels must be given training to enable them to play their part in a systematic and professional manner.' (1987)

It may be useful to consider what others have done before setting out to design our own programmes. Although we may each feel that we work in a unique situation we should beware of reinventing the wheel. There are certain elements which we feel are vital in any such programme and we will indicate practical ways of dealing with these later in the chapter.

The World Health Organization

The WHO from its regional office for Europe has been involved in a number of ventures; these are related to its work on 'Targets for Health for All' and in particular to target 31 that 'by 1990 all member states should have built effective mechanisms for ensuring quality of patient care within their health care system'. In October 1984 a consultative group met to 'begin preparing guidelines for the setting of standards and to create a slide/tape presentation and two pamphlets to stimulate interest among nursing groups'. These aids were then used by the nurses in the participating countries to assess their effectiveness in raising awareness. It became clear that there was some difficulty in understanding the terminology being used. It was also necessary for members of the group to spend time themselves learning to set standards in a workshop setting before they felt confident to return to their respective countries and teach others. It is a sad fact that we in this country do sometimes expect nurses to be able to write standards for their own practice with sometimes little or no guidance.

In the following year (1985) the WHO European Office set up a working group 'to discuss and make recommendations on training in quality assurance in both basic, post-graduate and continuing education as well as different categories of health personnel.' The aim of their educational programme was to improve the knowledge, skills and attitudes of nurses in quality assurance of health care. They were encouraged in their work by the fact that it seemed to fit in well with the work of introducing the nursing process and of using nursing norms. To those in this country whose experience of introducing the nursing process has not been singularly successful this may not be good news.

This group produced a model curriculum with information about curricular content, methods for evaluation and strategies for introducing quality assurance into the curriculum.

The United States of America

Nurses in the United States have been involved in introducing quality assurance for much longer than their colleagues in Europe. In the early 1970s the Rush-Medicus system was introduced in Chicago by Hegyvary and Haussmann. A large focus of their educational programme in introducing their quality monitoring instrument was on the preparation of the observers and coordinators who would initially test it out and subsequently put it into practice.

Orientation workshops were set up to 'familiarize nurse-observers with the quality monitoring instrument and to train them in its use.' It was emphasized that not only was their attendance necessary but the attendance of the coordinators was also required so that they would know what the observers were looking for and also to 'gain an appreciation of the criteria on which quality scores would be based.' Coordinators were members of staff who were chosen to be responsible for all study activities in the hospital and would act as a focus for communication in the process of quality monitoring.

The intention of these workshops was to develop significant inter–observer reliability and this is obviously a key feature in the development of any such scheme. To recap, inter–observer reliability is defined as the level of agreement among observers, meaning, what percentage of the time two or more observers collecting data from the same source at the same time agree on what they observe. Each observer was required to complete identical worksheets for the same patients and their responses were compared. Haussmann et al. (1976) report a 90% success rate for the workshops which is indicative of its level of success. Each of the workshops followed a similar pattern and included:–

1 Introduction and overview of the project and methodology.
2 Data collection procedures focusing specifically on scheduling observations: randomly selecting patients for review: checking patient classifications: hospital policies that related to specific evaluation criteria and with which observers . . . had to become familiar; review of records regarding care, e.g. Kardex, nursing notes.
3 Review and discussion of criteria in the master list, particularly those that required interpretation and judgement.
4 Trial use of quality work sheets.
5 Testing for inter-observer reliability.

There is no doubt that the methods of Haussmann et al., could be used here without too much modification to meet the needs of a British instrument. The need to ensure that the method used is reliable is imperative wherever it is being used.

Our American colleagues have also emphasized the need to repeat the testing of Inter–observer reliability at least twice a year to ensure that the skills acquired are still effectively functioning.

The British scene

We have indicated in an earlier chapter that the introduction of general management has been one of the forces in the drive to implement quality assurance programmes in this country. It has therefore been in the second half of this decade that we have seen most impetus in the preparation of staff for their various roles in such a scheme.

Charles Shaw (1986) writing in the King's Fund publication 'Introducing quality assurance' acknowledges 'the urgent demand for ideas on implementing quality assurance''. This publication was 'an attempt to summarize the basics' on this subject and included the important area of teaching and learning for quality assurance.

There is an acknowledgement that all health personnel need an introduction to the subject, but at that stage (1986) in its introduction the need was greatest amongst those officers at district level whose specific responsibility quality assurance was. They set out the elements of a training programme in terms of objectives which we quote here as we believe that they are a useful starting point in looking at such a programme.

Knowledge –	of the significance of quality assurance
	of principles and methods of quality assurance
	of existing activities/structures and their potential
	of existing sources of data/information
	of specific examples of quality assurance in practice
Attitudes –	that quality is identifiable and achievable
	that quality can be improved
	that quality is everybody's business
Interpersonal Skills –	to negotiate a local strategy
	to translate principles into local practice
	to implement change within organizations and among individuals
	to respect and develop staff contributions
	to teach/act as catalyst for all health disciplines
	to handle the 'poor performer'
Technical Skills –	to collate data from financial, administrative and clinical sources
	to design and implement local surveys and research
	to evaluate results of surveys and research
	to use common coding systems required for the interpretation of managerial and clinical statistics
	to use performance indicators on microcomputers
	to present information succinctly and clearly.

This initiative at national level has been taken up by other bodies at a more local level. An example of this can be found in the programme put out by the Oxford Health Authority in 1987. Although organized by Oxford they invited participants from other health authorities. The courses were designed for senior, middle and first-line managers who had an interest in quality and who would be involved in local initiatives.

Their programme included a planning and resourcing workshop for those people at district level who would be directly concerned with the setting up of a quality assurance programme. There was also a workshop on the concept of quality circles which would be helpful to those wishing to introduce this at local level and very importantly a specific course to prepare those who would act as facilitators and equip them with the skills they would need to do this successfully.

Other courses were also concerned with particular aspects of quality circles and there were two courses designed to tackle customer skills and problem-solving skills respectively. These are areas which are obviously part of a programme to improve quality but may not be seen as essential in initially getting a scheme off the ground. They are undoubtedly areas were nurses do need more expertise and should be considered as part of an overall educational package associated with improving quality of care.

An interesting approach to the introduction of quality assurance at district level is described by Griffiths (1988). This was a decision made by the Durham Health Authority to make use of Action Learning Sets initially at district and then at unit level. These action sets were used in relation to a number of managerial problems but were of particular use in getting to grips with the concept of quality and the introduction of ways of looking at standards of care.

It would be inappropriate to examine the use of action learning sets in depth in this book, however, the concept is a useful one and it is worth outlining the process here.

Action learning is a method of problem-solving which also offers scope for personal learning and development. In the case of the manager, he/she prepares to take action on the job – and at the same time learns about him/herself as a manager and as a person. An action learning set is usually a group of four to seven managers who meet with a set adviser. In the case of the Durham group the set had a total of 11 members and included medical, para-medical staff, administrators and a ward sister. The advisor was either Robin Gourlay, of the International Medical Centres, or the District Psychologist.

The way that members of an action learning set can learn from experience can be illustrated as follows:

problem described/feelings shared
clarity/new perspectives ┊ gained from set counselling
options explored, ┊ one option chosen
intermediate action ┊ by problem holder
review of progress ┊ at a later meeting

The problem set by the District General Manager at Durham was 'to prepare guidance to enable managers and departmental heads to define standards for their services' and it was the intention that the set would work together for a period of about 12 months.

It is still early days in the working of this particular set to say how effective it will finally be, but already they report 'a greater understanding of quality assurance and action learning'. They have also produced an action plan and acknowledge that the way forward will be to create performance standards supported by relevant information systems.

The educational programme

This chapter so far has looked at work done by different groups working at a fairly high level, we would now like to consider what preparation nurses specifically need to ensure that the system for monitoring patient care is correctly initiated and works well.

We have described in Chapter 2 how a scheme may be set up and the key people who need to be involved. The district needs to have agreed its strategy, both as a general principle for the district, and its strategy in relation to nursing standards, and to have formulated an action plan. The Durham experience above is one way of achieving this. Part of such an action plan may be the identification of the roles of those who will be critical in the implementation phase. This is a point made by Sale (1988) writing about the work done by West Dorset in standard setting.

Sale identifies three groups of nurses whose role needs to be established, or identified in relation to a quality assurance programme. These include the district coordinator, the facilitators and that of the nurse manager. Once those roles are clearly identified then appropriate educational programmes need to be set up to ensure that they are prepared to act effectively in these roles.

The role of the district coordinator may involve:−

- developing a framework for standard setting
- training facilitators
- supporting and advising facilitators
- chairing the district steering group

Preparation for this role may necessitate the individual attending one of the national or regionally organized programmes as described above or this may be done on a local basis, either by initiating an action learning set as indicated previously or by the district setting up workshops or conferences and inviting in outside experts.

The role of the facilitator is a major one in the success of a scheme. It may involve:

- acting as a source of advice and support for colleagues
- teaching colleagues to write and monitor standards of care
- liaising with the district coordinator

It is vitally important that an effective educational programme is set up locally to ensure that this key person is well prepared.

Those chosen to be facilitators must first themselves have shown an interest in quality and have high standards in their own practice.

Workshops should be set up to cover three main areas:

1 To provide the knowledge base from which they will operate.
   This comprises the principles, theory and practice of setting, writing, and monitoring standards.
   It must include adequate opportunity to write standards so that they feel confident to do this themselves before attempting to teach others.
2 To enable facilitators to develop the inter-personal skills which will prepare them to teach and advise others
   a) working with groups and group dynamics. This is essential in order that they may be able to work effectively as group leaders, to understand what is happening in the group, and to be able to influence group activities

b) teaching skills. This group may already have had some experience of the theory and practice of teaching in either basic or post-basic courses: one must not assume such previous experience and in any case it may be necessary to familiarize facilitators with any teaching aids that are proposed as part of the educational programme that they may be expected to use.

In many districts nurses in clinical areas are setting their own standards of care. This is important, as we have said earlier, because in doing so they have to think through their own expectations of care and once set they then have a clear feeling of ownership which is so important if they are to be achieved. One difficulty we should bear in mind is the need to have consistency in the way standards are written when a number of groups are involved. Writing standards is no easy task, the success of such work depends on the ability of the facilitators in clinical areas to pass on their skills to others. This only serves to underline the need for strong educational input for facilitators.

The manager must also be aware that her role must now encompass the monitoring and evaluation of standards. She will be required to understand and act on the results of monitoring exercises. Those who are acting as facilitators or monitors within her unit will also require her support; she must therefore be aware of their roles and responsibilities.

One of the most important roles is that of the person who uses the monitoring tool to assess whether or not standards are being met. This as we have suggested may be the responsibility of the facilitator but it may also be done by nurses who are specially selected and prepared for the role. These nurses need to be objective in their approach, a quality which requires judgements to be made without bias caused by personal values or beliefs. In any health district it is likely that there will be a number of people involved and it is crucial to the success of the scheme that there is inter–observer reliability. We mentioned earlier in this chapter the workshop set up by Haussmann et al. (1976) and we would certainly recommend that the content and teaching strategy which they employed be adapted for use here.

Neither must we forget those whose work will be under observation (either directly or indirectly) when nursing quality is assessed. It is important that their need for information is also taken into account when planning an educational strategy.

Vivien Jenkinson (1985) has suggested that they need to know:–

- what it is about – the aims, principles, benefits, risks
- what will actually happen – when, where, how, how often
- what answers can be expected – what format, frequency, acceptability, detail level
- what resultant actions might happen – education, re-training

How will these workers feel about the observations?
What defence mechanisms will they use?

It is important that people are informed about what is going to happen and how it will involve them; but initially the presentation of such material may be kept to essentials because, as Jenkinson points out: 'listening to people expressing their opinions after some experience can be even more important than telling them beforehand'. Therefore it is important to arrange rather longer sessions after auditing has been done to allow for the discussion that will inevitably take place. The role of the manager in these sessions is vital to ensure that the experience becomes a positive one and that people are supported when they may feel threatened.

In this chapter we have identified four specific areas of educational need. We do not wish to denigrate the skills of teachers who may be reading this book but we do feel that there may be those who have no formal educational background who may be expected to initiate a Quality Assurance programme and who may be grateful for some suggestions for workshop programmes.

What we have included here are all workshops which have been tried and tested elsewhere; we do not presume to suggest that these are the only effective methods, we merely offer them for your consideration.

Standard setting workshop

Aims

- To enable participants to understand the concept of quality assurance in health care; so that they may effectively participate in such activities in their own clinical area.
- To facilitate the setting of standards and criteria for the

evaluation of nursing care, and the development of a quality measuring instrument.

Objectives

Participants will be able to:–

Choose a conceptual framework suitable for standard setting in his/her practice

Write a standard for structure, process, and outcome which is applicable to his/her area

Write two criteria for each standard

List and discuss the necessary characteristics of a standard and criterion

Name two quality monitoring methodologies used by health professionals. Discuss their strengths and weaknesses.

Discuss the implications of designing an instrument to measure the quality of nursing care.

Outline of the day

Introduction to each other and to the programme

Without preparation each participant is asked to take five minutes and write a standard appropriate to his/her area of work. This is used subsequently to allow the participant to check learning during the day.

Presentation by workshop leader on
• What is quality assurance?
• The development of a quality monitoring methodology
• Definitions and examples of standards and criteria will be given.

Group work In groups of three to four people each participant will write a standard of his/her own choice. The group will then choose one of these standards and jointly write appropriate criteria for that standard. A leader will be chosen by the group who will present the work of the group to the others. Each presentation will be open to constructive criticism by the rest of the group.

Based on Kemp N. (1987)

Teaching skills workshop

Aim To enable nurses to maximize their teaching skills, feel more confident in a teaching role, and use teaching aids appropriately.

Objectives By the end of the workshop the participants will be able to:
• Analyse the concepts of teaching and learning
• Identify the role of the teacher
• Evaluate their present performance as a teacher
• Identify their personal learning needs to enable them to become more effective teachers
• Observe appropriate teaching methods, i.e. the 'talk', discussion groups
• Practise appropriate teaching methods in the 'safety' of the group
• Observe and practise the use of teaching aids, i.e. over-head projector, flip-charts
• Evaluate their own learning

Outline of workshop

Introduction to the workshop and to each other

Self assessment of present performance as teachers
Group discussion

'What is teaching, what is learning?'
Presentation by the group leader

'What do I need to learn to be an effective teacher?'
Identification of participants needs, setting objectives
Individual and small group work

'Planning a talk'
Presentation by the group leader

'Leading a discussion'
Presentation by leader followed by small group work

'Do I need teaching aids?'
Demonstration and practice using material produced by previous group work

Evaluation discussion of the workshop to identify learning which has taken place and how it happened.

This particular workshop works better if it can be spread over two days preferably one or two weeks apart to allow participants the opportunity to put some of their teaching into practice. This can then be used in the second day as a means of learning from experience.

Based on Hobbs W. and Staley M. (1986)

Group dynamics workshop

Aim To provide participants with an awareness of group dynamics, to explore leadership styles and to examine the functions of small groups.

Outcomes By the end of the workshop participants will be able to:

Identify the characteristics of groups and their prevalence in everyday life

Identify group processes and how these can help or hinder the decision making process

Understand the variety of roles which individuals may have in groups

Recognize the importance of listening skills in groups and the factors which contribute to and detract from effective listening

Identify a range of leadership styles and how these may be adapted or improved

Recognize the range of behaviours within groups which may cause difficulties

Use strategies to respond to difficulties while working with groups

Outline of the Workshop Introduction to the workshop
Establishing personal contact within the group
Negotiating the ground rules for the participants

The WHY of groups —
>   their characteristics and how they function
>   making them function better
>   decision making in groups

Individual roles in groups –
>   positive and negative roles
>   range of responses possible
>   importance of valuing contributions

Developing listening skills –
>   recognition of listening skills
>   value of effective listening
>   how do listeners respond?

Leadership styles –
>   to identify a range of styles
>   consider the effectiveness of a variety of styles
>   adapting and improving styles

Coping with difficult group members –
>   exploring what behaviours are difficult
>   developing strategies to cope
>   sharing skills and resources

How can we use these skills in our particular groups?

Evaluation of workshop

In conducting such a workshop the facilitator will himself be making use of the skills described. This makes for an experiential approach. Discussion and group exercises play a large part in such a course. It may also be more profitable to run this over two days despite the necessity to warm up on the second day.

Satow and Evans Working with groups TACADE, 2, Health Education Council, London.

Inter-observer reliability workshop

Aim To maximize the likelihood of obtaining high quality results from a quality monitoring exercise by improving the skills of those doing the audit.

Outcomes By the end of the workshop participants will be able to:
- Understand the methodology being used and the reasons for its choice

- Identify their part in the quality assurance programme for nursing
- Use the agreed instrument safely and with confidence
- Make records clearly and appropriately
- State with confidence their interpretation of standards and criteria as used in their auditing area

Outline of the Workshop Introduction and overview of the quality assurance programme.

Background to the choice of monitoring instrument. The monitoring instrument – time must be spent familiarizing participants with all aspects of this and in particular how they are expected to use it.

Standards and criteria – discussion of interpretation of these to ensure no areas open to doubt

Data collection procedures – using patient records
interviewing techniques
recognition of acceptable evidence
use of manual (if appropriate)

Recording results This is a participatory workshop and time must be spent ensuring that everyone has the opportunity to question and resolve any problems they may have. The use of the instrument needs to be tested rigorously to ensure reliability. This needs to be assessed by having participants complete identical audits on the same patient and comparing responses. Haussmann et al. (1976) reports a 90% agreement on such comparisons by the end of the workshop! Should we be content with any less?

Based on Haussmann et al., 1976.

References

Gaunt R., Kendall R. (1985) Action Learning – a short manual for set members, Greater London Employers Secretariat and Brent Libraries (GLES), Alembic House, 93 Albert Embankment, London SE1.

Griffiths W. (1989) Action Learning for Quality Assurance – A Diary. *International Journal for Health Care and Quality Assurance* vol. 1 no. 1 29–31.

Haussmann R. K. B., Hegyvary S. T. (1976). Field testing: The nursing quality maintaining methodology; phase II. *Nursing Research.* Sept/Oct 1976 **25**(5), 324–331.

Hobbs W., Staley M. (1984) Teaching Skills for Senior Nurses. Unpublished Work, Salisbury.

Jenkinson V. (1985) Preparation of Workers and Managers. Workshop at the King's Fund Centre 5, 6, 7, March 1985.

Kemp N. (1987) Developing a Quality Measuring Instrument for Practice – The Application and the Reality, Workshop programme to develop Standards and Criteria for the Evaluation of Care, Service and Performance. Unpublished work.

Kemp N. (1987) Quality Assurance Programmes in North America. Unpublished Report. Smith and Nephew – Florence Nightingale Scholarship Report. London: Florence Nightingale Committee.

Oxford Regional Health Authority (1987) Training for Quality. Regional Personnel Department, Oxford Regional Health Authority, Old Road, Headington, Oxford.

Report from a Working Group on Training for Quality Assurance of Health Services, Italy 25–28 June 1985. Nursing/Midwifery in Europe WHO – Regional Office for Europe vol. 3, no. 1, Mar. 1986.

Sale D. (1988) Down Dorset Way, *Nursing Times*, July 13, vol. 84, no. 28, 1988.

Saton A. and Evans M., Working with Groups TACADE, 2, Mt. St., Manchester. M25 NG.

Shaw C. (July 1986) Introducing Quality Assurance: King's Fund Project Paper. King Edward's Hospital Fund for London, 1986.

Summary report from the World Health Organization, Regional Office for Europe: second consultative meeting on the development of standards of nursing practice, Brussels, Belgium, 10–13 June, 1986. *Journal of Advanced Nursing*, 1987, **12**, 147–8.

Index